Nursing:
Concepts of Practice

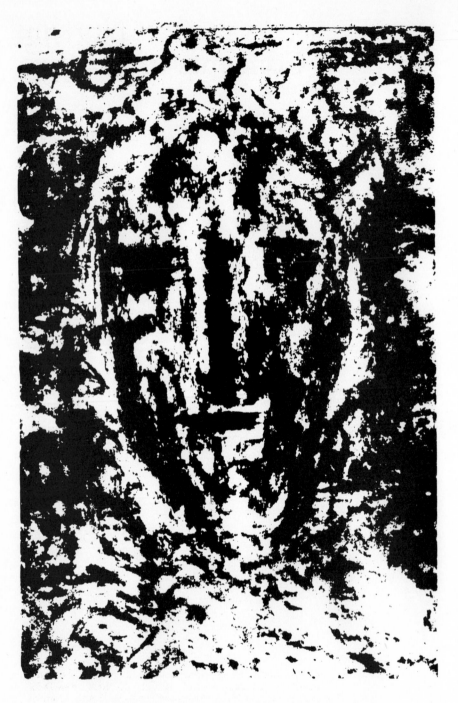

The Changing Face of Man. Original drawing by Walene E. Shields.

Nursing: Concepts of Practice

Second Edition

Dorothea E. Orem
Orem and Shields, Inc.
Chevy Chase, Maryland

McGraw-Hill Book Company

New York   St. Louis   San Francisco   Auckland   Bogotá   Hamburg
Johannesburg   London   Madrid   Mexico   Montreal   New Delhi
Panama   Paris   São Paulo   Singapore   Sydney   Tokyo   Toronto

This book was set in Times Roman by Offset Composition Services, Inc.
The editor was David P. Carroll;
the cover was designed by Mark Rubin;
the production supervisor was Carol Swain.
R. R. Donnelley & Sons Company was printer and binder.

NURSING: CONCEPTS OF PRACTICE

67890 DODO 83

Library of Congress Cataloging in Publication Data

Orem, Dorothea Elizabeth, date
    Nursing.

    Bibliography: p.
    Includes index.
    1. Nursing—Philosophy. I. Title.
RT84.5.073 1980   610.73   79-17289
ISBN 0-07-047718-3

Contents

Preface

The second edition of *Nursing: Concepts of Practice* is a result of the effort
expended by the author since 1958 to give form and structure to knowledge
that describes and explains nursing. This effort has been supported by the
convictions that nursing can and should be developed as a discipline and
that, in justice, persons enrolled in programs of nursing education should
be helped to become students of nursing or nursing scholars while they are
striving to develop the art of helping others through nursing.

The nursing student or scholar must be motivated to obtain insights
about the *domain* and *boundaries of nursing* as a health service in society,
to understand the *object of nursing* (that which the nurse takes cognizance
of and attends to as a nurse), and to become able to *think nursing* when
confronted with the complex and changing conditions of nursing practice.
The health care problems that individual nurses and their patients must
solve are becoming increasingly complex. Nurses must select and apply
nursing knowledge as well as knowledge from many different nonnursing
disciplines in order to understand the health care problems of individuals,
families, and communities. It is a nurse's mastery of key, organizing

nursing concepts that influences his or her selection and use of knowledge in a wide range of nursing situations. These key nursing concepts also influence the kind of information a nurse will seek in practice situations, how the information will be organized, and what meaning will be attached to it.

Nurses are coming to recognize that an item of information about a patient may have one meaning for a physician but quite a different meaning for a nurse. Every nurse and nursing student who aspires to practice nursing effectively must understand the nursing meaning of the range of human phenomena encountered in nursing practice. The nurse's role in relation to patients is now emerging from the obscurity imposed by an overemphasis on the relationship between the physician and the nurse and between the employing institution and the nurse. This emergence has been aided by the interests and concerns of nurses for the formalization of the processes and technologies of nursing practice, including the principles, theories, and rules of practice on which they are based. It is these principles, theories, and rules that help nurses to attach nursing meaning to the particular conditions and events of real nursing practice situations.

This second edition of *Nursing: Concepts of Practice,* like the first, is based on a general concept or theory of nursing that explains the relation of the nurse to persons or groups under nursing care. The theory has been used by nurses to guide their nursing practice endeavors and to extend and structure nursing knowledge. The concepts within the theory provide a conceptual framework of value to both nursing students and nurses who are developing as nursing scholars and practitioners. The mastery of the concepts should enable nursing students and nurses to place in perspective other descriptions of nursing, including those in areas of nursing specialization.

The ideas of nursing students and nurses who have used the first edition in its various stages of development have contributed in no small way to the present work.

Dorothea E. Orem

Nursing and Society

PREREQUISITES FOR NURSING

Although nursing is a valued service in many social groups, it is frequently in short supply for those who need it. A critical factor is the availability ratio: the number of persons in diverse places who require nursing at the same time and the deployment of nurses in relation to those persons. Nurses, as designers and providers of nursing, should be aware of indexes of the objective need for, the demand for, and the supply of nursing.

On a communitywide basis, it is a continual struggle to bring together those who can benefit from short- or long-term nursing and those persons who are able and willing to design, put into operation, produce, and manage systems of nursing assistance. This problem is or should be a concern of social groups that offer nursing as a community service.

A related problem is financing the provision of nursing in social groups. How much does it cost to produce effective nursing for those who need it? How should these costs be distributed within social groups? These questions have not been answered adequately in the United States, where for decades available nursing was produced in large part by nurses-in-training. This practice has changed, but the problem of financing nursing remains partly unaddressed.

Other prerequisites include (1) contact and communication among those who can benefit from nursing and those who are able and willing to produce this service; (2) willingness on the part of those who can benefit from nursing (or others who can legally act for them) and on the part of nurses to enter into and maintain legitimate interpersonal relationships in their respective positions of nurse's patient and nurse; and (3) interpersonal relationships that foster an understanding of how and to what degree nurses' patients can be helped through nursing. These three prerequisites for the production of nursing emphasize a requirement for the social legitimacy of the nurse-patient relationship, a mutual agreement to enter into such a relationship, and the purpose and, therefore, the limits of the relationship.

Effecting Nurse-Patient Relationships

Contact and communication among persons who can benefit from nursing and persons able and willing to provide it define the first prerequisite for the provision of nursing. Social groups have provided and continue to provide ways and means to effect this contact.

People generally come into contact with nurses in one of two ways: either they find nurses who publicly represent themselves as being engaged in the private or joint practice of nursing, or they come in contact with nurses through a health care institution that employs nurses. These two methods differ in terms of the way agreements are established and the number and nature of agreements among individuals and institutions. In the early and the middle years of this century, hospitals, state and district nurses' associations, and training schools for nurses maintained registers of nurses in private practice. These registers were the primary means of effecting nurse-patient contacts. Nurses would make their availability known by placing their names on a register, and individuals, families, or physicians whose patients needed nursing would contact nurses directly or through such a register. More recently, nurses have been maintaining their own offices, sometimes in group practice with other nurses or physicians, and this has made the office visit another method of effecting nurse-patient contacts.

In the second and more prevalent arrangement persons in need of nursing associate themselves with health care institutions, such as hospitals and visiting nurse associations, where nurses as well as other health workers are available. Under this arrangement nurses are usually employees of the institution as well as practitioners of nursing. Some of them, however, may be attached to registers.

Where nursing is provided in private or group practice, there is a contract or agreement between the nurse and the patient (or the patient's legal representative). Where nursing is effected through a health care institution, there is a contract or agreement between the patient and the institution. In this case, patients have contact with nurses who have been assigned to them by a manager or supervisor, who is usually also a nurse. Individuals who communicate with or accept care from assigned nurses indicate explicitly or implicitly that they agree to this relationship.

Nurses have not always been aware of the complexity of the relationships in the second arrangement. Nurses who are institutional employees should understand clearly that as members of a social group they occupy two social statuses: that of employee of a health care institution and that of nurse. This situation sometimes creates boundary maintenance problems and role conflict. The legal perspective in such situations is that the person who is the nurse in the status of *employee* is the *agent* (in the legal sense) of the employing institution. Figure 1-1 illustrates facets of this type of arrangement for nursing.

In both methods of bringing together nurses and persons who can benefit from their care, nurses may go where patients reside or patients may go to the location of the nurse. From this perspective, nursing as a service can be classified into four categories:

1   Home nursing—nurse goes to home of patient
2   Ambulatory nursing for adults—patient comes to location of the nurse (clinic or office) and returns home after the visit
3   Infant and child nursing in clinics or offices—patient is brought by parents or guardians to where the nurse is and returns home after the visit
4   Nursing for persons in any age group who are short- or long-term residents of health care institutions, such as hospitals or extended care facilities—nurses come to the institution where patients are in residence

Health care organizations such as medical centers with hospitals and health maintenance organizations may offer nursing services in all of these forms and locations.

From an occupational perspective nurses should accept nursing cases in accord with the fit between their individual nursing capabilities and the nursing requirements of those seeking nursing care. Determining whether individuals or groups evidence needs or requirements that nurses can legitimately meet is an essential nursing action. After this determination has been made, nurses should make a more detailed investigation of the nursing requirements of the individual or group. Finally, in light of a precise knowledge of their own nursing capabilities, nurses, as persons responsible for their own nursing acts, must make the judgment that they

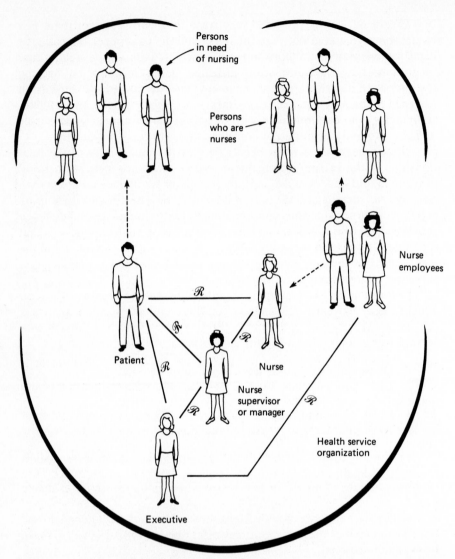

Figure 1-1 Nurse and patient relationships in health service organizations (R = relationship).

do or do not have the nursing capabilities required. If the nurse judges that he or she has the requisite capabilities, the nurse can enter into an agreement with the person seeking care (or those acting for the person) about the nature and form of the nursing that will be provided. At this point the nurse in private or group practice or the nurse who is an employee of a health care institution is in a position to negotiate with patients (or those acting for them) about the provision of nursing.

Development of Nursing Situations

The development of nursing situations requires that those who can benefit from nursing are willing to associate with and receive health services from particular nurses. Nurses must, in turn, be willing to maintain continuing contact and communication with these persons in order to provide nursing for them. The relationships of nurses to their patients and to others who are significantly related to the patient should develop into effective interpersonal relationships within which nursing needs can be determined and nursing can be produced.

Those in need of nursing and nurses may be unwilling to bring about or maintain the necessary conditions for nursing, or those who require nursing may be unaware that they have agreed to nursing when they contract for hospital care. Such individuals are surprised and unaccepting when nurses attempt to determine the characteristics of their nursing needs. On the other hand, persons who expect to receive nursing may be concerned and frightened when they are attended by aides, technicians, or orderlies and have no contact with nurses. Without a willingness on the part of nurses and patients to work together to accomplish nursing goals, nursing situations cannot exist. Ideally, nurses foster the development of mutual respect and trust in their relationships with their patients. They maintain the frequency of contact and the kind and amount of communication with patients and their families essential to determining and meeting patients' requirements for nursing.

NURSING AS HUMAN SERVICE

Nursing is made or produced by nurses. It is a service, a mode of helping human beings, and not a tangible commodity. Nursing's form or structure is derived from actions deliberately selected and performed by nurses to help individuals or groups under their care to maintain or change conditions in themselves or their environments. This may be done by individuals or groups through their own actions under the guidance of a nurse or through the actions of nurses when persons have health-derived or health-related limitations that cannot be immediately overcome.

When and why people can be helped through nursing, as distinguished from other forms of human service, is a critical question for nurses. The answer provides nurses with a knowledge of the proper focus of their efforts in social groups, indicates the boundaries of nursing practice, and identifies the object of nursing knowledge, the subject matter areas of nursing, and the domain of the nursing sciences. Without knowledge and understanding of the proper object of nursing, nurses cannot identify those with whom they can have a legitimate nursing relationship.

In modern society, adults are expected to be self-reliant and responsible for themselves and for the well-being of their dependents. Most social groups further accept that persons who are helpless, sick, aged, handicapped, or otherwise deprived should be helped in their immediate distress and helped to attain or regain responsibility within their existing capacities. Thus, both self-help and help to others are valued by society as desirable activities. Nursing as a specific type of human service is based on both values. In most communities people see nursing as a desirable and necessary service.

Historical works and the investigations of anthropologists provide evidence that, in the past, societies recognized the social position of nurse and provided ways and means to have nurses. In some situations, persons became nurses because of their position in the family or in the larger society. In other situations, individuals were recruited to become nurses, as is presently done in many countries. Preparation for nursing was both formal, through prescribed systems of training, and informal. Modern society introduced science-based education preparatory to nursing practice. The continued presence of active nurses in a society indicates that nursing is a desired and utilized service.

What is nursing? What are the nurse's contributions to the health and well-being of individuals, families, and communities? Is it to give care? Is it to bring about psychological adjustment so that a person will be able to accept and to live with illness or disability and develop personally, utilizing his or her human potential? Is it to be a helper to the physician by implementing prescribed measures of care for the patient? What nurses do can be considered as providing an affirmative answer to each question. However, the answers do not adequately describe how and why nursing is specifically different from other human services.

Every human service has a special concern for some aspect of human functioning or daily living that defines what the service does and thus differentiates it from other services. Nursing has as its special concern *the individual's need for self-care action and the provision and management of it on a continuous basis in order to sustain life and health, recover from disease or injury, and cope with their effects.* Self-care is a requirement of every person—man, woman, and child. When self-care is not maintained, illness, disease, or death will occur. Nurses sometimes manage and maintain required self-care continually for persons who are totally incapacitated. In other instances, nurses help persons to maintain required self-care by performing some but not all care measures, by supervising others who assist patients, and by instructing and guiding individuals as they gradually move toward self-care.

When do nurses enter into the life situations of individuals in support of their self-care actions? Societies specify the conditions that make it legitimate for its members to seek the various kinds of human services that are provided. These conditions become the criteria that members of the society use in determining whether or not a particular human service can or should be used. The condition that validates the existence of a requirement for nursing in an adult is *the absence of the ability to maintain continuously that amount and quality of self-care which is therapeutic in sustaining life and health, in recovering from disease or injury, or in coping with their effects.* With children, the condition is the *inability of the parent (or guardian) to maintain continuously for the child the amount and quality of care that is therapeutic.* The word *therapeutic* is used to mean supportive of life processes, remedial or curative when related to malfunction due to disease processes, and contributing to personal development and maturing.

Requirements for nursing cannot be met unless they are recognized. Physicians identify the need for and seek nursing for their patients. Friends and family members also may recognize when a person needs nursing, and adults may recognize their own needs for assistance. The family is often the first line of assistance when its members are in need. When family, friends, or neighbors are unable or unwilling to help, assistance with management or maintenance of self-care may be sought from organized nursing services. Nursing may be provided in the home or in health care institutions on an inpatient or outpatient basis. There may or may not be a sufficient number of nurses to provide the needed service. Organization for the delivery of nursing service is a need of every community.

Physicians traditionally have had as the focus of their service the health and disease states of individuals. Their concern is with life processes, body structure, and interferences with life and developmental processes. Physicians evaluate health states, determine evidence of the presence or absence of disease, and prescribe and give therapy to maintain health and to cure or control disease or the effects of injury and disease. When able, persons under medical care are expected to manage their own health affairs and maintain the type of self-care they require. When unable, assistance from persons other than the physician is required. Nursing is required whenever the maintenance of continuous self-care requires the use of special techniques and the application of scientific knowledge in providing care or in designing it.

It is an accepted practice for the physician to see patients periodically. The time a physician spends with a patient varies with the patient's health state and the medical care techniques utilized. Some patients see their physicians once a year, once a month, or more frequently. Physicians do not remain continuously with chronically ill or disabled patients. In the event of serious injury or when life processes or rational processes have been seriously interfered with, the physician may remain with patients for prolonged periods, sometimes working closely with nurses and other health care workers. Patients, nurses, and other specialized workers carry out measures of care prescribed by the physician, and nurses and others assist patients in preparing for measures of care to be performed by physicians. In such instances, a person's self-care becomes linked not only to the medical care given by the physician but also to care or services given by other health personnel, sometimes working as a team. Nurses must often synthesize or unify a variety of care elements into a process of self-care action for the patient.

Nursing as a human service has its foundations, on the one hand, in persons with needs for self-care of a positive, therapeutic quality and limitations for its management or maintenance and, on the other, in the specialized knowledge, skills, and attitudes of persons prepared as nurses. Societies must provide ways and means to bring individuals in need of nursing into relationships with qualified nurses. These relationships should be sustained as long as specialized techniques of care are required or until the person or a family member becomes able to manage and maintain the required self-care. Nursing, therefore, has foundations that can be conceptualized as biological, behavioral, and social.

NURSE AND PATIENT ROLES IN SOCIAL GROUPS

Individuals who receive help and care from persons qualified as nurses are referred to as *nurses' patients* or *clients*. The terms are used interchangeably to symbolize the social status and roles of persons under the care of nurses. From a sociological perspective, the terms *nurse* and *nurse's patient* (or *client*) signify related statuses or positions in social groups. Each status carries with it a *role,* that is, a set of prescriptions for organized action through which the status is filled. Nurses must be aware of the professional-occupational prescriptions for their roles as nurses and the role prescriptions for nurses and patients that are part of the general culture of social groups. General cultural prescriptions about nurse and nurse's patient roles may vary from one social group to another. The specific understandings individual nurses and those under their care have about their roles operate as underlying assumptions about the expectations and actions of the nurse and the nurse's patient in each nursing situation.

In real nursing situations, nurse's patient roles are specified by the reasons why the nursing is required and by what can and should be done under prevailing conditions. Nurses can help their patients to know and fulfill their roles only when nurses themselves know why and how their patients can be helped through nursing. Nurses' roles become specific in actual nursing situations by their knowledge of why and how an individual, singly or as a member of a family or group, can and should be helped through nursing.

Status and Role

The sociological concept of *status-role*, when combined with an understanding of when, why, and how people can be helped through nursing, can aid nurses in their efforts to develop insights about the *fit* or the *relatedness* of their actions to those of patients. A nurse's domain of action within a nursing situation may extend to some or to all or nearly all matters related to the existence and functioning of those under nursing care. How many aspects of the patient's daily life are encompassed in the nurse-patient relationship indicates the *extensity* of the relationship. The extensity of nurse-patient relationships varies with the patient's capabilities for self-care. For example, the extensity of a nurse-patient relationship is great when persons under nursing care have little or no capability for self-care because of their health state and the health-related nature of their continuing self-care requirements. This is so because nurses' roles extend to and encompass matters related to the moment-to-moment existence of such individuals.

The *intensity* of a nurse-patient relationship reflects the meaning that nurse and patient attach to their role relations. A nurse, for example, may know that nursing care can facilitate a patient's movement toward relative self-sufficiency in self-care. The patient, on the other hand, may view some types of help proffered by the nurse as intrusions into his or her life, or a patient may fear to be alone and may desire a nurse's presence continually, or a patient may dread being in the physical presence of a nurse who is rough or verbally abusive. Ideally, in adult nursing situations the extensity as well as the intensity of a nurse-patient relationship has an objective basis in (1) the patient's self-care abilities, limitations, and potential for action and (2) the meaning that nursing care has in relation to the patient's current and future well-being and to the nurse's effectiveness in filling the status of nurse.

Nurses at times have misconceptions about the rights and responsibilities of those who are seeking or who are under nursing care. The nurse-patient relationship is contractual in nature. This means that the functions and responsibilities of nurses are necessarily limited to matters within the domain of nursing, that the help sought is for a limited time, and that nurses are remunerated (directly or indirectly) for the help provided. There should be an initial agreement between the nurse and the nurse's patient or between the nurse and those responsible for the patient's affairs about the general characteristics of the nursing required and the nursing to be provided. The responsible person may be the parents of a child, the legal guardian of an adult, a person with the power to act for an adult, or the next of kin. At times executives of health care institutions employing nurses may need to be informed about these agreements. As previously indicated, each nursing situation requires that nurses must establish that persons or groups who have been represented to them as being in need of nursing are indeed in need of it and that they, as nurses, are able and willing to provide nursing. When nurses are employees of health care institutions, such as public health organizations, hospitals, or nursing homes with which patients have contracts for care, there should be a second, preferably explicit, verbal agreement between the nurse and each patient or individuals acting for the patient about the nurse's willingness to provide nursing and the patient's willingness to receive nursing from assigned nurses. Patients and their families should be informed about the goals to be sought through nursing.

Ideally, in health care institutions, explicit verbal agreements about the nursing to be provided should be made by the nurse who has diagnosed the particular patient's nursing requirements, who has designed a system of nursing assistance, and who bears continuing responsibility for nursing the patient. A number of nurses may contribute to the provision of nursing according to the original or adjusted design; this contributory care includes continuous observation of the patient. These nurses as well as the patient should know their own roles in addition to the role of the nurse who bears nursing responsibility for the patient. Nurses should understand that nursing requirements cannot be met unless they are known. Such knowledge comes only through directed and controlled observation, which necessitates contact and communication with the patient.

Agreements to provide nursing to individuals, families, or groups bind nurses to the provision of nursing in accord with objective nursing requirements. Nurses may be aware that they are not capable of providing the amount and kind of nursing required. At other times they are capable but know that external conditions, including the number of persons requiring nursing, will sometimes preclude the provision of sufficient nursing. When such conditions predominate, nurses, as responsible members of a social group, must be able to represent the existing situation prudently to the patient, to the employing executives, or to their own supervisors by indicating how all involved can best contribute to ensuring the safety and well-being of the patient. Nurses too often remain silent about situations where nursing is inadequate in quality or quantity or where patients have no contacts with nurses but are charged for it. One problem related to nursing charges within health care institutions results from the failure of those institutions to compute the costs of nursing for persons with differing nursing requirements. For example, the cost of nursing in some hospitals has been and continues to be included in a blanket charge for room accommodations. In some instances such charges are made when no nursing has been provided. Health care administrators sometimes seek to keep costs down by employing vocationally trained workers rather than nurses. When it is inadequately designed and planned, nursing can be a very costly service.

The relation of nurse to patient is a *complementary relationship*. This means that nurses act to help patients assume responsibility for their health-related self-care by (1) making up for existent health-related deficiencies in the patients' capabilities for self-care and (2) supplying the necessary conditions for the patients to withhold, for therapeutic reasons, the exercise of their capabilities or to maintain or increase their capabilities for self-care in order to maintain, protect, and promote their functioning as human beings.

The complementary nature of nurse-patient relations is a core concept in a nurse's development of insights about nursing and its practice. It is also the reason why nurses and patients or those who act for patients should seek to develop cooperative working relationships. Individuals, families, or groups under nursing care may be receiving other forms of health care, for example, medical care from one or more physicians, sometimes accompanied by a vast array of paramedical services. A nurse's patient, more likely than not, will be in contact and communication with relatives, friends, and work colleagues. The complementary nature of nurse and patient roles is also manifested by nurses' contacts with others who are significant to their patients and who represent a range of statuses.

Nurses require insights about conditions that militate against cooperative working relationships. For example, nurses should seek to understand the cultural elements involved in the prejudicial attitudes or discriminatory practices of social groups. These elements may affect both nurses and patients in their role fulfillment. Such elements include the prevailing attitudes of members of a social group regarding skin color, national origin, religion, degree of affluence and influence, social status, social deviance, or even being male or female. Such cultural elements can influence how nurses help patients in the development or exercise of their self-care abilities.

Patients too are influenced by such factors and may be reluctant or initially refuse nursing care or care from particular nurses. If nurses are to become safe and successful practitioners they must learn to deal with their own prejudices and discriminatory practices. They can learn to recognize such attitudes in their patients, help patients express their difficulties, and at times move to an early resolution of problem situations.

Role-Set

The sociological concept *role-set* can add an essential dimension to nurses' understanding of the complexity of the nurse role in some nursing situations. The term *role-set* stands for the idea that each status, for example, that of nurse or nurse's patient, involves the status-holder not in a single role but in a set of roles that may include contact with persons in other social statuses. The totality of roles is known as the set of roles associated with a specific status.

The concept of role-set, which is associated with a specific status and role, must be distinguished from that of *multiple roles*. For example, a person qualified in a society as a nurse may act to provide nursing care to patients. In addition, this person may also assist physicians in their performance of medical care measures for patients, or may function as a medical care technician, a clerk, or a manager of a total system of health service. The fact that, historically, nurses in health care institutions have had multiple roles has tended to obscure their central role of providing nursing to those in need of it. The fact that nurses have performed, and in some settings continue to perform, in the roles of physicians' assistants, medical care technicians, clerks, housekeepers, or managers does not make these roles nursing practice roles. This is because they involve nonnursing activities outside the domain of nursing practice. In organizations, however, combining a number of roles into one organizational position is common.

A related consideration in nursing is that the majority of nurses in health care institutions are employees as well as nurses. The role-set associated with the status of employee differs from the role-set associated with the status of nurse. Nurses' and their employers' failures to recognize the differences in these roles and to effect a legitimate alignment of them have hindered the progress of health care institutions and those nurses who are employed in them.

Nurses' patients as well as nurses may be operating concurrently within a number of other statuses and roles. Nurses and their patients may experience role conflicts in trying to fulfill the responsibilities of two or more roles. For example, a nurse's patient who is also a mother may find that fulfilling her responsibilities to herself for health-related self-care conflicts with her homemaking role and the role expectations she holds for her husband and children with respect to contributing to the conduct of the household. Persons under nursing and medical care who are confronted with a need to change life-style in order to care for themselves may not be able to do so until they have attended to the pressing duties of another role, for example, occupational role. Nurses should become able to help patients who have the necessary capacities to work out methods to become free enough, and therefore responsible enough, to provide or to manage their own self-care. Nurses and patients must learn to recognize and resolve role conflicts in order for them to achieve general nursing goals.

THE PROBLEM OF VARIETY AND NUMBERS

In 1893 Florence Nightingale's descriptions of the "art of nursing the sick" and "health nursing or general nursing" were published and made available to nurses.[1] Nurses historically have served the sick and the well in a variety of settings. Nurses have worked in the homes of persons in need of nursing, in clinics, and in hospitals. They have worked with community groups and in industry in the interests of the prevention of injury and illness and toward the maintenance and promotion of desirable health states for individuals and communities. They have worked to improve sanitary conditions in hospitals. They were in the forefront of recognizing the importance of understanding the social and behavioral dimensions of health care and in caring for individuals based on a recognition of their uniqueness as persons.

It is questionable, however, whether nurses have adequately explored the problems of providing nursing in social groups in terms of (1) the variety of nursing requirements and (2) the numbers of individuals with a range of types of nursing requirements who need nursing at the same time in a number of locations. The problem of supplying the numbers of people who need or want a service is a perennial problem in all human services. But the combined problem of numbers of people and varieties of requirements is the perennial problem of the health care services.

The problem of providing sufficient nursing to meet the demand for it is of great significance for nursing. Individual nurses, particularly in health care institutions where patients are in residence, may have responsibility for many patients during the same time period. This is stressful for both patients and nurses. It is a situation that demands the nurse's exercise of high-level planning skills in order to develop creative designs for the production of nursing.

The ability of nurses to creatively design adequate means for identifying and describing nursing requirements and to design, put into operation, and manage systems of nursing assistance for individuals, families, and groups is one characteristic of the *professional* nurse. Throughout nursing history there has been an inadequate number of nurses who could function to achieve these goals (for a number of reasons). The author believes that nurses have not operated with the insight that nursing, like other arts and sciences, has a proper object or focus; traditionally, nurses were trained to relate to individuals or groups under nursing care in order to (1) perform standardized nursing care measures for them and (2) socialize patients to institutional regimens to which nurses and patients

---

[1] Florence Nightingale, "Sick Nursing and Health Nursing," in Isabel A. Hampton et al. (eds.), *Nursing of the Sick 1893*, McGraw-Hill, New York, 1949, pp. 24–25.

were expected to conform. For many years nurses-in-training were not helped to envision care for individuals, families, and specific groups within nursing populations. How to look at people from a nursing perspective continues to be a problem in nursing circles. This problem will not be resolved until nurses are able and willing to ask and answer the question: when and why can people be helped through nursing as distinguished from other forms of health care?

The interest in nursing theories exhibited by nurses in the late 1970s is one indication that they may be approaching that stage of development where many more of them will become able to take an objective nursing approach toward the practice of nursing. For too long nurses have been unable to make the *nursing dimensions* of their practice explicit, even though some nurses have been and are able to make explicit other dimensions of nursing situations, such as public health, medical, psychological, or sociological dimensions. More nurses have been able to perform discrete nursing tasks than to "think nursing" within particular situations of practice. Nurses will become able to make explicit the nursing dimensions of their practice as they conceptualize more and more fully the proper object of nursing in social groups and use their concepts in the practice of nursing.

Nursing is action. The term *nurse* considered as a verb, an action word, is defined in dictionaries by the use of the noun *nurse*—for example, "to act as or be employed as a nurse." A nurse is identified as one trained to care for and wait upon the sick, injured, or infirm under the direction of a physician. Medicine is identified as a science and an art concerned with the prevention, cure, and alleviation of disease. Nursing will never be publicly recognized as science and art until nurses are able to explain why some people need and can benefit from nursing at particular times. Without such an explanation there is no basis for the development of nursing science and for the proper formation of individuals in the art of nursing.

Nurses for too long have used the medical sciences and physicians' medical orders for their patients as the primary underpinnings of nursing practice without expression of the nursing foundation. The medical sciences are important in supplying nurses with one type of required knowledge. Validated nursing knowledge, however, indicates how nurses should use medical and other sciences in their conceptualizations and in their work. If nurses concern themselves only with what physicians order for their patients who are also under nursing care these patients would sometimes be in dire straits. For decades enlightened nurses and physicians have understood the differences between *nursing care* and *medical care* and have been able to generalize about the probable points of articulation between these two human services and to identify actual points of articulation between nursing and medicine in particular health care situations. These nurses and physicians have a basis for communication and collaboration to meet objective requirements for coordinating their actions in the interests of patients who are under both forms of health care.

If they are to design solutions to the problem of providing nursing to numbers of people with a range of nursing requirements, nurses must begin to develop nursing science. Such sciences would include descriptions and explanations of when, why, and how people can be helped through nursing as well as validated rules of nursing practice. Nursing science would not deal with all aspects of human affairs but with carefully defined aspects of it, referred to as the "world of the nurse."

ROLE COMBINATIONS

The primary work of nurses is to provide nursing in accord with the needs people have in assuming responsibility for their health-related self-care. The practitioner of nursing, the nurse, is the designer and provider of nursing in the social group. Nurses cannot become and remain competent practitioners, however, unless they know and are able to apply nursing and nursing-related knowledge in their practice. This knowledge is being continuously formulated and validated through the work of nursing theorists, researchers, and the developers of nursing technologies, techniques, and rules of practice. The status and role of nurse therefore should be linked always to that of *student of nursing* and *student of nursing-related disciplines*. Too many nurses remain intellectually impoverished in their chosen field in an age characterized by explosions of knowledge in the health care disciplines and the disciplines related to them. Any man or woman entering nursing should understand the essentiality of combining the status and role of nursing practitioner with that of nursing student or scholar. The dual role is necessary for the adequate provision of nursing in this period.

Individuals cannot develop themselves as practitioners of nursing and as students of nursing without teachers. Some members of the nursing profession elect to teach nursing students. Ideally, teachers of nursing are prepared and are advancing in proficiency as nursing practitioners while becoming advanced scholars in one or more areas of nursing and in one or more nursing-related disciplines. Some teachers of nursing have not advanced themselves as nursing scholars. It is difficult, if not impossible, for nurses and nursing students to develop as scholars in a field as new as nursing science when they are without adequate guidance from advanced nursing scholars.

Because of the type of education they elect and the forms of nursing practice in which they choose to become proficient, nurses contribute to nursing in different ways. Nurses who function in the roles of nursing theorists, researchers, developers of nursing technologies, and teachers should be contributing to the advancement and further development of present and future nursing practitioners. The role of *developer* should be afforded greater recognition in nursing. It is the nurse developer who translates the findings of nursing science researchers into a nursing practice frame of reference. This is done by inventing processes, technologies, techniques, artifacts, and rules and by determining their effectiveness and reliability in practice settings. At times, developers invent valid and reliable ways of doing things and only later are the scientific foundations of these new practices identified.

NURSING EDUCATION

Schools of nursing have proliferated in the United States since the first schools were opened in the year 1873. Nursing education during the early period of its development was promoted by interested lay or professional people often associated with hospitals. Pioneer schools of nursing were modeled at least in part after the Nightingale School associated with Saint Thomas's Hospital in London,[2] which was opened in 1860 under the sponsorship of Florence Nightingale and financed through the Nightingale Fund.[3] Since World War II, nursing has entered the so-called scientific age in its history. Education for nursing has expanded to include a broader base in general studies, in the humanities and behavioral and social sciences, and in leadership and management. Traditional biological and medical science content remains in nursing programs, sometimes with considerable expansion and restructuring of emphasis.

With the ever-increasing knowledge of humanity and the complexity of health care and medical technology, there has been a concomitant demand for nurses prepared at the university level. In addition, the enactment of social legislation (Medicare and Medicaid) has greatly increased the need for nurses and for personnel to assist them in providing and managing nursing. The number and types of workers who serve by providing self-care assistance has increased rapidly since 1940. Not all workers are prepared or licensed as nurses. Some persons with minimal knowledge and skills work without supervision from nurses. Nurses are limited by external and internal factors in what they can do to meet nursing requirements in a community. Limiting factors include time, prevailing conditions, interests, values, and abilities of the nurses of a community. Effective organization of nursing services is essential both in the provision

[2]Mary M. Roberts, *American Nursing*, Macmillan, New York, 1954, pp. 7–19.
[3]Cecil Woodham-Smith, *Florence Nightingale, 1820–1910*, McGraw-Hill, New York, 1951, pp. 225–238.

of nursing and the maintenance of satisfaction among nurses. Modern nurses are no less capable than nursing leaders of the past. Finding ways to meet and keep up with changing requirements for nursing is the task of and a challenge to each nurse. Nurses have a substantial part in the process of moving communities toward standards of nursing practice that ensure safe and effective nursing. No other group can perform this task for nurses. Nurses, collectively, have a responsibility for the quality of the services they provide in a community.

Members of the younger generation of nurses have an education that has been enriched with modern science and technology and general studies. The young nurse may be in the formative stage of the art of nursing, but his or her foundation for its development may exceed that of nurses with years of nursing experience. Techniques and practices in current use are evaluated and sometimes questioned by younger nurses and nursing students. This is the role of each new generation, for in this way nursing practice is refined and enriched. Practices, since they tend to become fixed or institutionalized, are not easily changed, but without developmental change stagnation and deterioration of nursing effectiveness occur. Young nurses and nursing students should seek knowledge of valid but unrecorded nursing techniques from more experienced nurses who have attained nursing wisdom from thoughtful and effective nursing practice. Nurses who have developed techniques and have evidence of their effectiveness should contribute this information to the developing body of nursing knowledge. Identifying, validating, and recording techniques of nursing practice are important tasks in the continued development of a body of nursing knowledge.

Educating nurses for limited roles in nursing has been introduced in the United States. This is done in other fields and is a mark that a service is being extended to more and more persons. The content and length of programs of nursing education vary according to the roles for which different types of nurses are being prepared. In the delivery of nursing in communities and in institutions the contribution that each type of nurse is to make to nursing should be defined, and provision should be made for coordinating efforts in the interests of both patients and nurses. Division of the work of nursing among several types of nurses without providing for the coordination of effort and results leads to chaos. The demand for nurses who are effective in appraising the needs of individual patients for nursing and in designing systems of nursing assistance is increasing, along with the demand for nurses who can effectively supervise nurses who are prepared for limited roles. Changes in nursing education and changes in nursing practice are interrelated.

Nurses must be able to fill their positions in a spectrum of health care services developed around technologies of health care and health care problems. The nurse is not a solitary worker. The days when only physicians and nurses made up health teams is over. Expansion of the spectrum of health services places demands on nurses for coordinating actions with persons from an increasing number and variety of health services. The specific character of nursing activities will be closely related to the kinds of health problems that prevail in the community. For example, communicable disease, serious injuries from industrial accidents, and chronic illness result in needs for different types of nursing actions. Communities vary in the combinations of health problems that prevail, although certain health problems are common to all communities. The character of nursing activities is also affected by the way in which patients can be helped. The requirements of persons who are ill and are patients in hospitals or nursing homes sometimes result in heavy demands for continuing care by nurses and other types of personnel. Community health centers and health maintenance organizations brought an increased demand for nursing that emphasizes guidance and instruction in therapeutic self-care and help to patients so that they can identify and work with internal and environmental conditions that interfere with their self-care actions. Some industrial and business firms now employ nurses on a full-time basis to serve their employees' health needs. These nurses may give direct assistance to employees as the need arises, but they are primarily concerned with preventive measures related to the health and well-being of the firm's employees and their families. Many governmental, health, and welfare agencies also employ nurses in a variety of health-related activities. Regardless of the kinds of health and other problems that determine the specific work of the nurse, he or she is always recognized as a specialized worker with a distinctive social position and pattern of behavior. It has been indicated that the nurse's role in society focuses on (1) the maintenance of those self-care activities that individuals continuously need to sustain life and health, recover from disease and injury, and cope with the effects of disease and injury and (2) self-regulation of the individual's self-care capabilities.

CONCLUSION

Several general statements concerning nursing practice are made as a conclusion to this chapter. The statements may stimulate thought or discussion of nursing as a human service:

1 Nursing relationships in society are based on a state of imbalance between the *abilities of nurses to prescribe, design, manage, and maintain systems* of therapeutic self-care for individuals and the *abilities of these individuals or their families to do so.* The imbalance is in the direction

the nurses' abilities exceed those of other individuals. When the imbalance is in the opposite direction or when there is no imbalance, there is no valid basis for a nursing relationship.

2   Nursing practice has not only technological aspects but also moral aspects, since nursing decisions affect the lives, the health, and the welfare of human beings. Nurses must ask, "Is it right for the patient?" as well as "Will it work?"

3   Solutions proposed to problems of the management and maintenance of therapeutic self-care for patients and families with limitations on maintaining their own care may give rise to other problems, solutions to which may be difficult if not impossible.

SELECTED READINGS

Nursing

Bullough, Vern L., and Bonnie Bullough: *The Emergence of Modern Nursing*, 2d ed., Macmillan, New York, 1969.

Nursing Development Conference Group: "Selected Concepts of Nursing in the Public Domain," in *Concept Formalization in Nursing: Process and Product*, 2d ed., Little, Brown, Boston, 1979.

Philosophy

Plattel, Martin G.: *Social Philosophy*, Duquesne University Press, Pittsburgh, 1965.

Social and Interpersonal Situations and Communication

Allport, Gordon W.: *The Nature of Prejudice*, abr. Anchor Books, Doubleday, Garden City, N.Y., 1958.

Hall, Edward T.: *The Silent Language*, Anchor Press, Doubleday, Garden City, N.Y., 1973.

Hanson, Robert C., and Mary J. Beech: "Communicating Health Arguments across Cultures," *Nursing Research,* vol. 12, Fall 1963, pp. 237–241.

Haugen, Einar: "The Curse of Babel," *Daedalus*, vol. 102, Summer 1973, pp. 47–57.

Hays, David G.: "Language and Interpersonal Relationships," *Daedalus*, vol. 102, Summer 1973, pp. 203–216.

Larsen, Sister Paula A.: "Influence of Patient Status and Health Condition on Nurse Perceptions of Patient Characteristics," *Nursing Research*, vol. 26, November-December 1977, pp. 416–421.

Lewis, Garland Kathryn: *Nurse-Patient Communication*, 3d ed., William C. Brown, Dubuque, Iowa, 1978.

McCusker, Sister M. Peter: "Gracias, Dinora," *American Journal of Nursing*, vol. 72, February 1972, pp. 250–252.

Sowell, Thomas: "Ethnicity in a Changing America," *Daedalus*, vol. 107, Winter 1978, pp. 213–237.

Human Services

Chase, Richard B.: "Where Does the Customer Fit in a Service Operation?" *Harvard Business Review*, vol. 56, November-December 1978, pp. 137–142.

Demone, Harold W., Jr., and Dwight Horshbarger: *A Handbook of Human Service Organizations*, Behavioral Publications, New York, 1974.

Schulberg, Herbert C., Frank Bonker, and Sheldon A. Roen (eds.): *Developments in Human Services*, vol. 2, Behavioral Publications, New York, 1975.

Health Care—Delivery, Costs, Expenditures

Brickner, Philip W., et al. "Outreach to Welfare Hotels, the Homebound, the Frail," *American Journal of Nursing*, vol. 76, May 1976, pp. 762–764.

Dean, Andrew G.: "Population-Based Spot Maps: An Epidemiologic Technique," *American Journal of Public Health*, vol. 66, October 1976, pp. 988–989.

Hatcher, Gordon H.: "Canadian Approaches to Health Policy Decisions—National Health Insurance," *American Journal of Public Health*, vol. 68, September 1978, pp. 881–889.

Hu, Teh-wei (ed.): *International Health Costs and Expenditures*, U.S. Department of Health, Education, and Welfare, Public Health Services, National Institutes of Health Publication (NIH) 76-1067, Washington, D.C., 1972. Especially Chapter 2, Robert Maxwell, "International Health Costs and Expenditures—An Hors D'Oeuvre," pp. 3–21.

Jonas, Steven, et al.: *Health Care Delivery in the United States*, Springer, New York, 1977. Especially Chapter 5, Nancy R. Barhydt, "Nursing," pp. 96–119.

Keaveny, T., and Roger L. Hayden: "Manpower Planning for Nurse Personnel," *American Journal of Public Health*, vol. 68, July 1978, pp. 656–661.

Malany, Janet: "The Difference It Makes," *American Journal of Nursing*, vol. 72, February 1972, pp. 276–279.

Milio, Nancy: "A Framework for Prevention: Changing Health-Damaging to Health-Generating Life Patterns," *American Journal of Public Health*, vol. 66, May 1976, pp. 435–439.

Nursing in the World Editorial Committee: *Nursing in the World. The Needs of Individual Countries and Their Programmes*, The International Nursing Foundation of Japan, Tokyo, 1977.

Parker, Alberta W., Jane M. Walsh, and Merl Coon: "A Normative Approach to the Definition of Primary Health Care," *Milbank Memorial Fund Quarterly*, vol. 54, Fall 1976, pp. 415–438.

Sociology

Biddle, Bruce Jesse, and Edwin J. Thomas (eds.): *Role Theory: Concepts and Research*, Wiley, New York, 1966.

Hardy, Margaret E.: *Role Theory: Perspectives for Health Professionals*, Appleton-Century-Crofts, New York, 1978

Litman, Theodor J.: "The Sociology of Nursing," in *The Sociology of Medicine and Health Care: A Research Bibliography*, Boyd and Fraser, San Francisco, 1976, pp. 134–157.

Merton, Robert K.: *On Theoretical Sociology*, Macmillan, New York, 1967, pp. 39–45.

Shils, Edward: "The Academic Ethos," *The American Scholar*, vol. 47, Spring 1978, pp. 165–190.

Sorokin, Pitirim: "Familistic, Contractual, and Compulsory Relationships and Systems of Interaction," in *Social and Cultural Dynamics*, rev. and abr., Porter Sargent, Boston, pp. 436–452.

Yarmolinsky, Adam: "What Future for the Professional in American Society?" *Daedalus*, vol. 107, Winter 1978, pp. 159–174.

Law

Creighton, Helen: *Law Every Nurse Should Know*, 3d ed., W. B. Saunders, Philadelphia, 1975.

Rothman, Daniel A., and Nancy Lloyd Rothman: *The Professional Nurse and the Law*, Little, Brown, Boston, 1977.

Nursing Practice and Nursing Knowledge

COMPLEMENTARITY OF NURSING KNOWLEDGE AND PRACTICE

Nursing students and nurses entering practice want to learn to perform nursing effectively and satisfactorily for themselves and their patients. Since nursing is offered to the public as a help or service, nurses should attain and maintain a high level of nursing knowledge and nursing performance, but to be effective in practice nurses must gain nursing knowledge before they enter practice. Nurses also must have and use knowledge from a number of nursing-related fields. It is reasonable to expect that all nursing students will be introduced to nursing as a field of knowledge as well as a field of practice.

Levels of Nursing Knowledge

Nursing knowledge describes and explains individuals and groups from the perspective of the incapacitating conditions that prevent them from effectively meeting known requirements for self-care or the care of dependents. Nursing knowledge also describes and explains how people can be nursed. It can be organized into distinct nursing sciences when the objects of nursing inquiry are identified and made explicit. What nurses have subjected to verification and have communicated to colleagues and students through published works or verbally constitutes the body of nursing knowledge that should be available to students of nursing. One of the essentials for the continued existence and for the growth and development of nursing as a human service is the systematic development of nursing sciences. Nursing knowledge has degrees of generality, ranging from knowledge that is generalizable to any and all nursing situations to knowledge that is specific to a particular instance of nursing practice.

Figure 2-1 indicates levels of the generality of nursing knowledge. Level 1 signifies knowledge generalizable to all instances of nursing. Level 2 signifies less general knowledge, illustrated in Fig. 2-1 by three hypothetical types of nursing cases. Level 3 knowledge applies to a subtype of nursing case. Level 4 signifies a particular instance, a case, a concrete occurrence of requirements for nursing where characterizing conditions exist at specific values. The term *case* is used to mean a situation in which an individual or a group can be helped through nursing. Knowledge at Levels 1, 2, and 3 is presupposed for nursing practice as well as for nursing research. Acquiring Level 4 knowledge is an essential component of nursing practice; in nursing research, acquiring Level 4 knowledge constitutes the data collection phase of research focused on instances when nursing is required.

General Nursing Knowledge

Nursing knowledge that can be generalized to all instances of nursing includes general, comprehensive theories of nursing. Those general theories that demonstrated validity and reliability provide the conceptual structure for the development of the nursing sciences. Figure 2-2 illustrates the comprehensive theory of nursing expressed in Chapter 1. The con-

Nursing knowledge
Descriptive and explanatory of:

1 Nursing cases, undifferentiated	$x, x, x, \dots\dots\dots\dots\dots\dots\dots\dots\dots, x^n$		
2 A range of types of nursing cases	xy, xy, xy	xz, xz, xz	xzy, xzy, xzy
3 Subtypes of cases		xza, xzb, xzc	
4 A particular instance, a case		xzb (existent at specific values)	

Figure 2-1   A representation of nursing knowledge by degrees of generality.

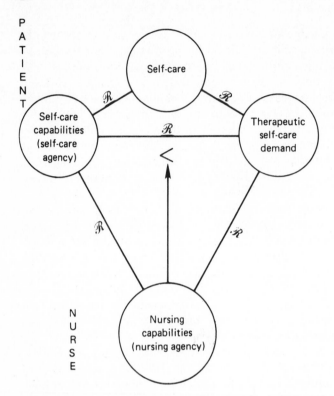

Figure 2-2 A conceptual framework for nursing (R = relationship; < = deficit relationship, current or projected).

ceptual elements and their relationships shown in Fig. 2-2 are aids to understanding the logic of nursing. Mastery of these elements should aid nursing students in thinking nursing, in organizing empirical data and ideas, and in communicating nursing facts and ideas to patients and others.

The conceptual elements shown in Fig. 2-2 constitute one essential aid (but not the only one) for nurses who want to (1) know what to attend to and observe in nursing practice situations; (2) develop appropriate nursing imagery, for example, about what will occur if nursing is not provided when particular conditions exist; (3) characterize and name what is observed; (4) attach human and nursing meaning to what is observed; and (5) know the range of possible courses of action that are open to nurses and patients in a range of nursing situations.

The mastery of a general, comprehensive *theory of what nursing is* and *why nursing is produced and supported by social groups* is a first step for nurses who want to be aware of the relationship between what they know and what they do as nurses. Thinking nursing and seeing and conceptualizing the whole situation in a particular nursing situation is distinct from viewing nursing as the skilled performance of a standarized set of tasks. Task performance is a constituent of all practical endeavors, and nurses must be skilled in task analysis, in task synthesis to form valid courses of action, and in task performance. Nurses should understand how tasks, including task sequences, fit into the larger designs for self-care and nursing and understand how to select and perform those tasks. Rationales and contraindications for task selection should be understood. Furthermore, nurses must know the performance capabilities required if they are to perform tasks effectively.

Nursing Practice

The domain of nursing practice can be described in terms of the populations who can be helped through nursing. Candidates for nursing are those with *deficit relationships* between (1) their current or projected capability for providing self-care or dependent care and (2) the qualitative and quantitative demand for care. The reason for the deficit relationship between care capabilities and care demand is associated with the health state or health care needs of those requiring care (see Chapter 1). For example, parents who are competent to provide effective child care for their 6-year-old son may not be competent care providers if their son sustains multiple injuries in an accident or undergoes a severe life-threatening episode of viral pneumonia. In both situations the child requires medical care and nursing; nursing actions would be adapted to the child as an individual, to the child's health state, to the child's age and particular state of development, and to the diagnostic and treatment measures prescribed by physicians.

The domain of nursing practice can also be described in terms of the activities in which nurses engage when they provide nursing. The author has identified five areas of activity for nursing practice:

1 Entering into and maintaining nurse-patient relationships with individuals, families, or groups until patients can legitimately be discharged from nursing
2 Determining if and how patients can be helped through nursing
3 Responding to patients' requests, desires, and needs for nurse contacts and assistance
4 Prescribing, providing, and regulating direct help to patients (and their significant others) in the form of nursing
5 Coordinating and integrating nursing with the patient's daily living, other health care needed or being received, and social and educational services needed or being received.

A model of the domain of nursing practice is thus a composite of persons characterized by conditions that generate nursing requirements and the actions that nurses perform when they provide nursing to these persons.

A GENERAL THEORY OF NURSING

The general comprehensive theory of nursing presented in broad outline in Chapter 1 and as a conceptual framework in Fig. 2-2 was first expressed by the author in 1958. Since then, it has been refined, used, validated, and further developed by the author, her colleagues, and others. The theory can be used by nursing students as a guide toward understanding nursing's domain and in identifying the conceptual foundations of nursing science. It is presented below in summary form.

Nursing theories are accounts (descriptions and explanations) of relationships and serve as plans or briefs to organize the outlook of nurses. They are the results of the theorist's creative ideas and of inquiry and investigation based on those ideas. Since one description or explanation in a field may be replaced by a richer and more unified view, theory development can be viewed as a process of understanding relationships and applying knowledge in practice or research situations. A nursing theory does not tell nurses what to do or what not to do; it does specify whether and under what conditions the existence of relations among events can be predicted and what relationships or conditions should be deliberately brought about in order to keep events within desired ranges.

The theory of nursing presented in Chapter 1 and shown in Fig. 2-2 is made up of three theoretical constructs:

1   The theory that *self-care deficits* and deficits for dependent care, when health-derived or health-related, are predictive of nursing requirements denotes the proper object or focus of nursing in social groups and provides criterion measures for identifying those who need nursing. It also explains when and why nursing is required.

2   The theory that *self-care* and dependent care are systematized, deliberate actions that, when continuously and effectively engaged in, regulate structural integrity, human functioning, and human development (sometimes through the control of environmental factors) explains why these forms of care are necessary for the continuance of life.

3   The theory that the product of nursing practice is a *nursing system*(s) through which the capability of patients to engage in self-care is regulated and self-care is continuously produced explains how persons can be helped through nursing.

Each of these three theories is discussed here in terms of its central or unifying idea, its theoretical propositions, and its underlying presuppositions.

The Theory of Self-Care Deficit (or Dependent-Care Deficit)

The Central Idea People can benefit from nursing because they are subject to health-related or health-derived limitations that render them incapable of continuous self-care or dependent care or that result in ineffective or incomplete care. This theory constitutes the core of the author's general comprehensive theory of nursing.

Propositions

1 Persons who take action to provide their own self-care or care for dependents have specialized capabilities for action.

2 The individual's abilities to engage in self-care or dependent care are conditioned by age, developmental state, life experience, sociocultural orientation, health, and available resources.

3 The relationship of individuals' abilities for self-care or dependent care to the qualitative and quantitative self-care or dependent-care demand can be determined when the value of each is known.

4 The relationship between care abilities and care demand can be defined in terms of *equal to, less than, more than.*

5 Nursing is a legitimate service when:

   a Care abilities are less than those required for meeting a known self-care demand (a deficit relationship).

   b Self-care or dependent-care abilities exceed or are equal to those required for meeting the current self-care demand but a future deficit relationship can be foreseen because of predictable decreases in care abilities, qualitative or quantitative increases in the care demand, or both.

6 Persons with existing or projected care deficits are in, or can expect to be in, states of social dependency that legitimate a nursing relationship.

Presuppositions The theory of self-care deficits elaborated above rests on a number of presuppositions. These presuppositions link the theory of self-care deficit to the theory of self-care and to the idea of nursing as one of the health services institutionalized by social groups.

SET ONE

1 Self-care is a form of self-management.

2 Self-care is necessary for life itself, for health, for human development, and for general well-being.

3 Self-care and the care of dependents rest on the cultural attainments of social groups and on the educability of their individual members.

SET TWO

1 Societies provide for the human state of social dependency by instituting ways and means to aid persons according to the nature of and the reasons for their dependency.

2 When they are institutionalized, the direct helping operations of

members of social groups become the means for aiding persons in states of social dependency.

3   The direct helping operations of members of social groups may be classified into those associated with states of age-related dependency and those not so associated.

4   Direct helping services instituted in social groups to provide assistance to persons irrespective of age include the health services.

5   Nursing has been and is one of the health services of Western civilization.

The Theory of Self-Care

The Central Idea   Self-care and care of dependent family members are learned behaviors that purposely regulate human structural integrity, functioning, and human development. The theory of self-care denotes the relationship between the deliberate self-care actions of mature and maturing members of social groups and their own development and functioning as well as the relationship of the continuing care of dependent family members to their functioning and development (see Fig. 2-3).

Propositions

1   Self-care and care of dependent family members are learned within the context of social groups by human interaction and communication.

2   Self-care and care of dependent family members are deliberate actions sequentially performed to meet known needs for care.

---

1   Select an individual (a relative, friend, or associate or an inpatient or outpatient at a hospital) who has a chronic disease, has sustained an injury, has experienced an acute illness, or is pregnant for the first time.

2   In accordance with the individual's ability, interest, and willingness to comply with your request for information, ask the following questions (rephrase if desired) and record the answers.

   a   Since the occurrence of (name the conditioning factor, disease, injury, etc.), do you have to care for yourself differently than you did before its occurrence?

   b   What are some of your new activities or tasks?   How did you learn about the need to engage in them?

   c   How do you fit the new tasks into the schedule of your daily activities?

   d   Can you do all of these new tasks for yourself?   If not, who helps you?

   e   Did you know how to do these new tasks before the occurrence of (same as in a, above)?

   f   How did you feel about learning to do the new tasks?   How do you feel about doing them now?

   g   Of all the things that you know you should do, are there some things that you tend to forget or deliberately decide not to do?   If so, why?

Figure 2-3   Exercise to assist in the development of a concept of self-care.

3 Requisites for self-care have their origins in human beings and their environments.

4 Some requisites for self-care are common to all human beings; others are specific to the developmental and health states of individuals.

5 Universal self-care requisites and ways of meeting them may be modified by the age, sex, or developmental or health state of individuals.

6 A specific process or technology (a way to achieve a purpose) or a specific set of processes or technologies is necessary to meet each self-care requisite.

7 Self-care (or dependent care) as a process or system results from the individual's deliberate use of conceptualized processes or technologies to meet known self-care requisites.

8 A system of self-care or care for dependent family members may be composed of courses of action to meet universal care requisites and requisites associated with developmental and health states.

9 Existing self-care or dependent-care systems are made up of the discrete actions individuals select and perform in sequence in order to meet their particular self-care needs.

10 Knowledge of actual self-care or dependent-care systems results from the deliberate recall and ordering of the discrete actions that were performed or from observing the care actions of others.

Presuppositions

1 All things being equal, human beings have the potential to develop their intellectual and practical skills and the motivation essential for self-care and care of dependent family members.

2 Ways of meeting self-care needs (self-care processes, technologies, and practices) are cultural elements and vary with individuals and larger social groups.

3 Self-care and care of dependent family members are forms of deliberate action, which is affected by an individual's repertoire of and his or her predilection for taking action under certain circumstances.

4 Identifying and describing recurring requisites for self-care and the care of dependent family members leads to investigating and developing ways to meet known requisites.

The Theory of Nursing System(s)

The Central Idea   Nursing systems are formed when nurses use their abilities to prescribe, design, and provide nursing for legitimate patients (as individuals or groups) by performing discrete actions and systems of action. These actions or systems regulate the value of or the exercise of individuals' capabilities to engage in self-care and meet the self-care requisites of the individual therapeutically.

Propositions

1 Nurses relate to and interact with persons who occupy the status of nurse's patient.

2 Legitimate patients have existent and projected continuous self-care requisites.

3 Legitimate patients have existent or projected deficits for meeting their own self-care requisites.

4 Nurses determine the current and changing values of patients' continuous self-care requisites, select valid and reliable processes or technologies for meeting these requisites, and formulate the courses of action necessary for using selected processes or technologies that will meet identified self-care requisites.

5 Nurses determine the current and changing values of patients' abilities to meet their self-care requisites using specific processes or technologies.

6 Nurses estimate the potential of patients to (*a*) refrain from engaging in self-care for therapeutic purposes or (*b*) develop or refine abilities to engage in care now or in the future.

7 Nurses and patients act together to allocate the roles of each in the production of patients' self-care and in the regulation of patients' self-care capabilities.

8 The actions of nurses and the actions of patients (or nurses' actions that *compensate for the patients' action limitations*) that regulate patients' self-care capabilities and meet patients' self-care needs constitute nursing systems.

Presuppositions

1 Nursing is a helping service.

2 Nursing is a complex form of deliberate action performed by nurses over some duration of time for the sake of others.

Summary

The theoretical constructs that constitute this general, comprehensive theory of nursing can serve nurses by giving a nursing focus to their endeavors in nursing practice and by providing a basis for organizing patient information. The concepts can also serve nurses in their endeavors to form the theoretical and the practical nursing sciences. The theories of self-care deficit, self-care, and nursing system(s) are further elaborated in subsequent chapters.

NURSING KNOWLEDGE AND NURSING EDUCATION

Nursing students can be helped to learn to think nursing in particular situations of practice when the following conditions exist:

1 Nursing is consistently represented and explained by nursing teachers and practitioners as having an objective field different from but sometimes touching or overlapping that of other health services. The nature and degree of this overlap is one index of the kind and amount of coordination that nursing will require with other fields. Skills in coordinating nursing with other forms of health care are developed within concrete situations of nursing practice.

2   Variations of the components of nursing are explicitly represented and explained in nursing courses. The relation of specific values of these components, either singly or in some combination, to the courses of action nurses can select from in providing nursing is described and explained.

3   The relationship of nursing theory and nursing questions to theory or areas of knowledge from nursing-related arts and sciences is made explicit by teachers of nursing.

The development of nursing programs to include nursing courses that contain explicit nursing knowledge is a major undertaking that needs the concerted and continued attention of advanced nursing scholars. In the broad field of nursing there are at least five disciplines of knowledge specific to nurses and nursing. The degree of development of the five disciplines varies but, currently, each discipline is developed to some degree. These five disciplines, named below, represent the author's effort to sort out the kinds of nursing knowledge offered in undergraduate nursing curricula and the kinds of knowledge essential for use in nursing practice.

1   Nursing's social field—dimensions of nursing as an institutionalized service in social groups under fixed and changing social, cultural, economic, and political conditions

2   Nursing as a profession and an occupation, including legal considerations

3   Nursing history

4   Nursing ethics

5   Nursing sciences

Each of the five disciplines is drawn upon to some degree in the development of undergraduate nursing courses. All five are essential, but the development and mastery of the *nursing sciences* are critical to nurses' continuing development and their attainment of the cognitional orientations essential to nursing practice. Figure 2-4 illustrates some of the focuses of forms of occupational education.

Because of the undeveloped state of the nursing sciences, the first edition of this book was conceived as a stopgap measure for introducing nursing students to theoretical constructs that could serve as guides to nursing practice. The theory of nursing presented in this chapter may be judged on first reading as being too abstract and therefore impractical for nursing practice purposes. Repeated use of the theory by nursing students

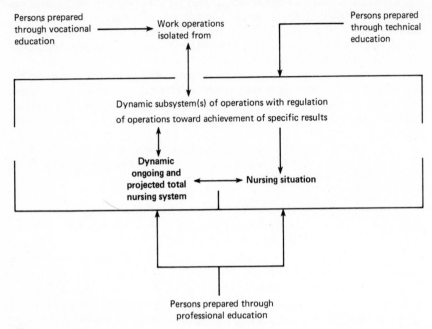

Figure 2-4 Focuses of forms of occupational education.

and practitioners, however, has demonstrated not only the theory's validity and reliability but also its utility in nursing practice. Mastery of the theory requires that individuals experience the theory in real nursing situations. This should be the goal of nursing students who seek to understand the central ideas and the propositions through which this theory of nursing is expressed. Subsequent chapters of this book will further develop the parts of the theory by relating the components of each to real conditions and events.

SUMMARY

Nursing has been explained as a response of human groups to one recurring type of incapacity for action to which human beings are subject, namely, the incapacity to care for oneself or one's dependents when action is limited because of health or health care needs. From a nursing point of view, human beings are viewed as needing continuous self-maintenance and self-regulation through a type of action named *self-care*. The term *self-care* means care that is performed by oneself for oneself when one has reached a state of maturity that enables him or her to take consistent, controlled, effective, and purposeful action. The unborn, the newborn, infants, children, the severely disabled, and the infirm cannot meet their own requirements for self-care.

Self-care, care of dependent family members, and nursing can be viewed within an ecological context as *human systems* formed from the interpenetrations of psychosocial and technological human systems. McHale refers to these humanly produced systems as an "external human metabolism."[1,2] The production of such human systems requires the capability for reflection and the genetic capabilities of "using symbols" and "assimilating human culture."[3] Diversity in human systems of infant and child care and care of the aged, the injured, and the infirm can be viewed as deliberate adaptations to the variety of the environments that members of social groups encounter or create. Nursing considered as a human system within social groups requires the presence and the actions of persons qualified as nurses. The status of nurse and that of nurse's patient require complementary roles for status fulfillment. The criterion measure for legitimacy as a nurse's patient is the presence of health-derived or health-related action limitations associated with the health state or health care needs of the person requiring care that render self-care or care of dependents impossible, incomplete, or ineffective.

Care of infants, children, the aged, and the infirm within social groups requires persons with knowledge and skills and the willingness to help others who are in need of direct personal care. Self-care and care of dependent members of social groups are adversely affected not only by the scarcity of material resources, such as food, but also by a lack of knowledge and skills and the absence of attitudes that foster the willingness to give of self by caring for others. Individuals who cannot give of themselves in aiding others tend to diminish themselves as persons.

SELECTED READINGS

Dickoff, James, Patricia James, and Ernestine Wiedenback: "Theory in a Practice Discipline, Part I. Practice Oriented Theory," *Nursing Research,* vol. 17, September-October 1968, pp. 415–435.

——, ——, and ——: "Theory in a Practice Discipline, Part II. Practice Oriented Research," *Nursing Research,* vol. 17, November-December 1968, pp. 545–554.

Ellis, Rosemary: "Characteristics of Significant Theories," *Nursing Research,* vol. 17, May-June 1968, pp. 217–222.

——: "Values and Vicissitudes of the Scientist Nurse," *Nursing Research,* vol. 19, September-October 1970, pp. 440–445.

[1]John McHale, *The Ecological Context: Energy and Materials,* World Resources Inventory, 1965.

[2]John McHale, "Global Ecology: Toward the Planetary Society," *American Behavioral Scientist,* vol. 11, July-August 1968, p. 30.

[3]Theodore Dobzhansky, *Genetics and the Origin of the Species,* 3d ed., Columbia University Press, New York, 1951, p. 304.

Giorgi, Amedo: "An Application of Phenomenological Method in Psychology," in A. Giorgi, C. T. Fisher, and E. L. Murray (eds.), *Phenomenological Psychology,* vol. 2, Duquesne University Press, Pittsburgh, 1975, pp. 83–103.

Glaser, Barney G., and Anselm L. Strauss: "The Purpose and Credibility of Qualitative Research," *Nursing Research,* vol. 15, Winter 1966, pp. 56–61.

McHale, John: "Man Plus," *Zygon,* vol. 6, September 1971, pp. 210–223.

Nursing Development Conference Group: *Concept Formalization in Nursing: Process and Product.* Little, Brown, Boston, 1979.

Plattel, Martin G.: "Philosophical Attitude," in *Social Philosophy,* Duquesne University Press, Pittsburgh, 1965, pp. 7–22.

Spellman, Susan: "Crohn's Disease: An Holistic Approach," in A. Georgi, C. T. Fisher, and E. L. Murray (eds.), *Phenomenological Psychology,* vol. 2, Duquesne University Press, Pittsburgh, 1975, pp. 130–139.

Zderad, L. T., and H. C. Belcher: *Developing Behavioral Concepts in Nursing,* Southern Regional Education Board, Atlanta, 1968.

Nursing and Self-Care

SELF-CARE

In the term *self-care,* the word *self* is used in the sense of one's *whole being.* Self-care carries the dual connotation of "for oneself" and "given by oneself." The provider of self-care is referred to as a *self-care agent.* The provider of infant care, child care, or dependent adult care is referred to by the general term *dependent-care agent.* The term *agent* is used in the sense of *the person taking action.* Self-care is the practice of activities that individuals initiate and perform on their own behalf in maintaining life, health, and well-being. Normally, adults voluntarily care for themselves. Infants, children, the aged, the ill, and the disabled require complete care or assistance with self-care activities. Figure 3-1 illustrates the concept of self-care and dependent-care agents.

Infants and children require care from others because they are in the early stages of development physically, psychologically, and psychosocially. The aged person requires total care or assistance whenever declining physical and mental abilities limit the selection or performance of self-care actions. The ill or disabled person requires partial or total care

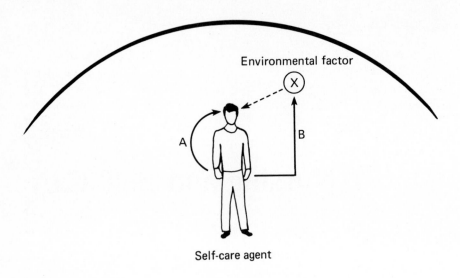

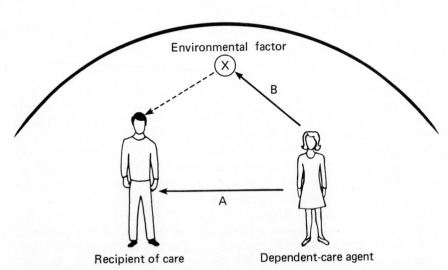

Figure 3-1 Self-care and dependent-care agents (A = care directed to self or to another who is the recipient of care; B = care directed to the regulation of environmental factors; X = environmental factor).

from others (or assistance in the form of teaching or guidance) depending on his or her health state and immediate or future requirements for self-care. Self-care is an adult's continuous contribution to his or her own continued existence, health, and well-being. Care of others is an adult's contribution to the health and well-being of dependent members of the adult's social group.

Self-care has purpose. It is action that has pattern and sequence and when it is effectively performed contributes in specific ways to human structural integrity, human functioning, and human development. The purposes to be attained through the kinds of actions termed self-care are named *self-care requisites.*[1] Three types of self-care requisites are identified: universal, developmental, and health-deviation. They rest on the following assumptions:

1 Human beings, by nature, have common needs for the intake of materials (air, water, foods) and for bringing about and maintaining living conditions that support life processes, the formation and maintenance of structural integrity, and the maintenance and promotion of functional integrity.

2 Human development, from the initial period of intrauterine life to the fullness of adult maturation, requires the formation and the maintenance of conditions that promote known developmental processes at each period of the life cycle.

3 Genetic and constitutional defects and deviations from normal structural and functional integrity and well-being bring about requirements for (*a*) their prevention and (*b*) regulatory action to control their extension and to control and mitigate their effects.

Self-care requisites as described here are generalizations about the purposes that individuals have or should have when they engage in self-care. Conceptualized self-care requisites that have been validated by their successful use in aiding individuals to manage their health and well-being become elements of the general culture or remain within the domains of the health care professions. Self-care requisites must be known before they can serve as the purposes of self-care. Universal self-care requisites should become known by all educable adults. Ideally, this also holds for developmental self-care requisites. For both types of requisites, however, reliable knowledge is not always effectively selected and adequately organized for public dissemination. Health-deviation self-care requisites usually become known by those who have genetic or constitutional defects or health deviations or whose family members or associates have such defects or health deviations.

When self-care requisites are viewed as formulated and expressed generalizations about the purposes of self-care, the ways and means

[1]In the first edition of the book, the term *self-care requirement* was used. *Requisite* is viewed as a more precise term. The practice of expressing requisites in terms of action was not followed in the first edition, although the nature of self-care requirements as purposes of self-care actions was explicit in their descriptions.

through which these purposes can be attained is an important consideration in understanding self-care as human action. For example, an adult who has been judged by herself and her physician to be edematous and in a state of fluid and electrolyte imbalance has, as one object of self-care, this health deviation self-care requisite: to maintain fluid intake at no more than 1000 ml during each 24-hour period. This is an adjustment of the universal self-care requisite to maintain a sufficient intake of water occasioned by the clinical observations and judgments of the physician. The actions to achieve this purpose must be known and be within the capabilities of the person with the self-care requisite (or another person who can act for the individual).

In addition to making judgments and decisions about the kinds of fluids to be ingested and the distribution of amounts over the 24 hours of the day, there are action sequences for procuring the fluids, preparing them as necessary for ingestion, measuring them into appropriate utensils, drinking them, and accounting for the fluids taken at particular times and for the entire 24-hour period. Throughout each 24-hour period there would be actions for self-restraint, self-orientation, and maintenance of awareness of the purpose of self-care. Acceptance of oneself as being in need of this kind of care (or at least willingness to attain the purpose of care) is also required.

The operations required to maintain fluid intake within a specified maximum may be thought of as a segment of a person's daily self-care. Since self-care directed to achieve a particular object is necessarily a series of actions performed in some sequence, self-care is properly referred to as an action system or a dynamic process. It is helpful for nurses and other care providers to conceptualize all self-care actions performed in sequence as constituting an individual's self-care system. Actions directed to meet particular, individual self-care requisites can be conceptualized as constituting subsystems of the total self-care system. The ways and means for meeting particular self-care requisites can be described in terms of (1) general method and (2) required operations or actions. In the example outlined in Fig. 3-2 the general method is drinking, the natural method used by human beings after infancy to consume substances in a liquid state. The sets of operations in Fig. 3-2 identify the kinds of actions to be taken to achieve partial results toward accomplishing one particular self-care purpose, using a specified method.

Required operations vary with general method. If the general method selected for use in the example in Fig. 3-2 was injection of fluids into a vein (intravenous administration of fluids), the types of operations required would conform in a general way to the sets named in Fig. 3-2 but the specific actions would differ. When the general method and required operations for achieving a type or range of purposes have been identified,

Particularized self-care requisite	General method	Sets of required operations
Maintain fluid intake at no more than 1000 ml every 24 h	*Ingestion by mouth,* drinking from a container	Seek and validate knowledge of the requisite, its meaning, its duration, and projected effects
		Prepare self, materials, and the environmental setting
		Consume measured fluids and account for the amounts consumed
		Monitor self for evidence of effects—desired or adverse
		Communicate results of monitoring to the prescribing physician

Figure 3-2 Elements of an action system to meet a particularized self-care requisite.

tested, and integrated into an explicit system of action, the result is a formulated process that becomes part of the technological knowledge of particular practice disciplines, for example, the intravenous administration of fluids.

Therapeutic Self-Care Demands

Nurses develop capabilities to (1) identify the self-care requisites of their patients, (2) select or confirm the general methods through which each identified requisite can and will be met, and (3) identify the actions to be taken in meeting each specific self-care requisite. Nurses should also develop their powers to identify and conceptualize not only specific self-care requisites, but also the totality of the demands for self-care action. The totality of self-care actions to be performed for some duration in order to meet known self-care requisites by using valid methods and related sets of operations or actions is termed the *therapeutic self-care demand*. An individual's self-care demand cannot be known until it is calculated. One result of effective nursing in some nursing situations is that patients become able to calculate their own therapeutic self-care demands, even persons who, because of limited movement, may not be able to execute some of the actions within the demand.

A therapeutic self-care demand is a humanly constructed entity, with an objective basis in information that describes an individual structurally, functionally, and developmentally. It has its theoretical base in the theory that self-care is a human function and in facts and theories from the human and environmental sciences. Formulating a therapeutic self-care demand requires investigating and understanding what self-care requisites exist and judging what can and what should be done. A therapeutic self-care demand is essentially a prescription for continuous self-care action through which identified self-care requisites can be met with stipulated degrees of effectiveness. Each person has requisites for self-care; to the degree that these are known and the ways for meeting them understood, individuals will experience demands for action to care for themselves (or dependent family members).

Practical and Therapeutic Aspects of Self-Care

Self-care action is practical in orientation. Performing a self-care measure involves a decision, a choice. This is so even with routine practices such as those related to food selection or personal hygiene. Unless self-care activities have become habitual practices, there is a need for reflection about what should be done and how it will be done. Knowledge of human functioning, one's present condition and circumstances, and known care measures provide a basis for such reflection. Some techniques for care in health and in illness are a part of the general culture. Others become known to individuals and families because of specialized education or practical experience in using the techniques. There is often a lag between developed techniques and their use. Available resources may affect the use of self-care techniques. Interests and motives are also determining factors. Individuals and families may adapt themselves to chronic ill health rather than learn about therapeutic care measures.

Self-care and care of dependents may be well intentioned but not therapeutic. It is necessary to determine the therapeutic value of practices prescribed by the general culture and even by health professionals. A single self-care practice or a whole system of self-care is therapeutic to the degree that it actually contributes to the achievement of the following results: (1) support of life processes and promotion of normal functioning; (2) maintenance of normal growth, development, and maturation; (3) prevention, control, or cure of disease processes and injuries; and (4) prevention of or compensation for disability. Some of these results are required by all persons on a continuing basis during all stages of the life cycle, but others are required only in the event of disease or injury.

Self-care is a practical response to an experienced demand to attend to oneself. The demands may originate in the individual, for example, a person experiencing a lack of energy or intense emotional reactions, or from knowledge that a care measure should be performed because it is health-promoting. Demands may originate from others, for example, the directives of parents to children or health workers to clients and patients or neighbors and friends. The demand as experienced is a stimulus to which the person responds in some manner. Demands may be met or ignored. Awareness of the demand may remain even when the demand has been ignored. A person may identify the presence of a tumor, knows he or she should seek medical assistance, but does not and yet worries about having cancer. When persons know that what they have experienced is significant to life or health, they feel a heavy responsibility toward themselves.

The self-care demands that all people experience and the demands experienced when there is illness, injury, or disability have two aspects: what is the purpose of requisite self-care and what is its nature? Self-care considered as a practical response requires answers to two questions: what is the nature of the demand and what action will constitute a therapeutic response to the demand?

Self-care requisites are expressions of the kinds of purposive self-care that individuals require. They should be expressed in terms of action, for example, "maintain a sufficient intake of water." Three types of self-care requisites were identified in the preceding section and are discussed here. Each type represents a category of deliberate actions to be taken by or for individuals because of their needs as human beings. Persons seeking understanding of self-care and self-care requisites will search for further descriptions and explanations of these requisites.

1 Universal self-care requisites are common to all human beings during all stages of the life cycle, adjusted to age, developmental state, and environmental and other factors. They are associated with life processes and with the maintenance of the integrity of human structure and functioning.

2 Developmental self-care requisites are associated with human developmental processes and with conditions and events occurring during various stages of the life cycle (e.g., prematurity, pregnancy) and events that can adversely affect development.

3 Health-deviation self-care requisites are associated with genetic and constitutional defects and human structural and functional deviations and with their effects and medical diagnosis and treatment.

When these three types of requisites are effectively met, they are productive of human and environmental conditions that (1) support life processes, (2) maintain human structures and human functioning within a normal range, (3) support development in accord with the human potential, (4) prevent injury and pathological states, (5) contribute to the regulation or control of the effects of injury and pathology, and (6) contribute to the cure or regulation of pathological processes. From the perspective of preventive health care, effectively meeting universal and developmental self-care requisites in well individuals is ideally in the nature of primary prevention of disease and ill health. Meeting health-deviation requisites may aid in the control of pathology in its early stages (secondary prevention) and in the prevention of defect and disability (tertiary prevention). Effectively meeting the universal and developmental self-care requisites is essential when there is pathology in order to maintain human structure and functioning and to promote development and thereby contribute to rehabilitation. Rehabilitation focuses on developmental self-care requisites associated with conditions resulting from pathology, medical diagnoses or treatment procedures, or the results of inadequate nursing or dependent care.

Universal Self-Care Requisites

Eight self-care requisites common to all human beings are suggested.

1 The maintenance of a sufficient intake of air.
2 The maintenance of a sufficient intake of water.
3 The maintenance of a sufficient intake of food.[2]
4 The provision of care associated with elimination processes and excrements.
5 The maintenance of a balance between activity and rest.
6 The maintenance of a balance between solitude and social interaction.
7 The prevention of hazards to human life, human functioning, and human well-being.
8 The promotion of human functioning and development within social groups in accord with human potential, known human limitations, and the human desire to be normal. *Normalcy* is used in the sense of that which is essentially human and that which is in accord with the genetic and constitutional characteristics and the talents of individuals.

These eight requisites represent the kinds of human actions that bring about the internal and external conditions that maintain human structure and functioning, which in turn support human development and maturation. When it is effectively provided, self-care or dependent care organized around universal self-care requisites fosters positive health and well-being. Table 3-1 presents general actions for meeting these eight requisites. The results of meeting each of the eight universal self-care requisites contribute in different ways to health and well-being.

The maintenance of sufficient intakes of air, water, and food provides individuals with the materials required for metabolism and energy production. The provision of effective care associated with elimination processes and excrements should ensure the integrity of these processes and their regulation as well as effective control of the materials eliminated. The maintenance of a balance between activity and rest controls voluntary

---

[2]Constituents of foods that human beings need are referred to as nutrients. These include proteins and the amino acids of which they are composed, fats and fatty acids, carbohydrates, minerals, and vitamins. Water is also a constituent of many foods.

**Table 3-1   General Sets of Actions for Meeting the Eight Universal
Self-Care Requisites**

1   Maintaining sufficient intakes of air, water, food
   a   Taking in that quantity required for normal functioning with
adjustments for internal and external factors that can affect
the requirement, or, under conditions of scarcity, adjusting
consumption to bring the most advantageous return to
integrated functioning
   b   Preserving the integrity of associated anatomical structures
and physiological processes
   c   Enjoying the pleasurable experiences of breathing, drinking,
and eating without abuses
2   Provision of care associated with eliminative processes and
excrements
   a   Bringing about and maintaining internal and external
conditions necessary for the regulation of eliminative
processes
   b   Managing the processes of elimination (including protection
of the structures and processes involved) and disposal of
excrements
   c   Providing subsequent hygienic care of body surfaces and
parts
   d   Caring for the environment as needed to maintain sanitary
conditions
3   Maintenance of a balance between activity and rest
   a   Selecting activities that stimulate, engage, and keep in
balance physical movement, affective responses, intellectual
effort, and social interaction
   b   Recognizing and attending to manifestations of needs for
rest and activity
   c   Using personal capabilities, interests, and values as well as
culturally prescribed norms as bases for development of a
rest-activity pattern
4   Maintenance of a balance between solitude and social
interaction
   a   Maintaining that quality and balance necessary for the
development of personal autonomy and enduring social
relations that foster effective functioning of individuals
   b   Fostering bonds of affection, love, and friendship;
effectively managing impulses to use others for selfish
purposes, disregarding their individuality, integrity, and
rights
   c   Providing conditions of social warmth and closeness
essential for continuing development and adjustment
   d   Promoting individual autonomy as well as group
membership

**Table 3-1   General Sets of Actions for Meeting the Eight Universal
Self-Care Requisites** (Continued)

---

5   Prevention of hazards to life, functioning, and well-being
   a   Being alert to types of hazards that are likely to occur
   b   Taking action to prevent the occurrence of events that may
      lead to the development of hazardous situations
   c   Removing or protecting oneself from hazardous situations
      when a hazard cannot be eliminated
   d   Controlling hazardous situations to eliminate danger to life
      or well-being
6   Promotion of normalcy
   a   Developing and maintaining a realistic self-concept
   b   Taking action to foster specific human developments
   c   Taking action to maintain and promote the integrity of one's
      human structure and functioning
   d   Identifying and attending to deviations from one's structural
      and functional norms

---

energy expenditure, regulates environmental stimuli, and provides variety, outlets for interests and talents, and the sense of well-being that comes from both. The maintenance of a balance between solitude and social interaction provides conditions essential for developmental processes in which knowledge is acquired, values and expectations are formed, and a measure of security and fulfillment is achieved. Solitude reduces the number of social stimuli and demands for social interaction and provides conditions conducive to reflection; social contacts provide opportunities for the interchange of ideas, acculturation and socialization, and the achievement of the human potential. Social interaction is also essential for obtaining the material resources essential to life, growth, and development.

Prevention of hazards to life, functioning, and well-being contributes to the maintenance of human integrity and therefore to the effective promotion of human functioning and development. The promotion of human functioning and development, in turn, prevents the development of conditions that constitute internal hazards to human life and to human functioning and development. It also promotes conditions that lead individuals to feeling and knowing their individuality and wholeness, to cognitional objectivity, and to freedom and responsibility as human beings. All eight requisites are interrelated. Some of these relationships are shown in Fig. 3-3. Understanding the relationship among requisites is important for nurses and other care agents. Care givers must ask and answer at least three questions in relation to the three self-care requisites of maintaining sufficient intakes of air, water, and food:

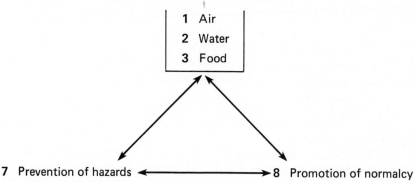

Figure 3-3   Interrelationships of some of the universal self-care requisites.

1   What is a sufficient intake of air, water, and food under known or hypothesized internal and external conditions? For example, should water and food intake be adjusted under conditions of heat stress and, if so, how?

2   What hazards, if any, are or may be associated with meeting each of these requisites for the intake of materials? How can identified hazards be eliminated or controlled? For example, the presence of noxious substances in inspired air, water, or food and food intakes that are not sufficient.

3   In meeting these three requisites for material intakes, can normal functioning and development be promoted and, if so, how? For example, by the institution and maintenance of patterns of food consumption based on a knowledge of the nutrients in consumed food, not just on habits and preferences.

To be effective the provision of care associated with elimination processes and excrements requires answers to the following:

1   What are the elimination patterns of individuals? Are current patterns congruent with former patterns?

2   What care practices or care measures are associated with acts of elimination and the disposal of excrements?

3   Do the identified elimination patterns or the care practices (or lack of same) in and of themselves constitute hazards?

4   What hazards, if any, are associated with preparation for or engagement in elimination under the individual's internal and external conditions?

5   What constitutes the norm for elimination for an individual? If elimination patterns are presently outside the norm, how can normal functioning be brought about?

6 What care practices related to acts of elimination and disposal of excrements would benefit individuals and the social group?

The provider of care in relation to maintaining a balance between activity and rest and a balance between solitude and social interaction would need to answer the following three questions:

1 What constitutes a balance between rest and activity and between solitude and social interaction under prevailing internal and external conditions?
2 What kinds and degrees of rest and activity or solitude and social interaction constitute a hazard under existing conditions?
3 What kinds and degrees of rest and activity or solitude and social interaction can be expected to maintain human structure and promote human functioning and development in relation to the human potential and its limits and at the same time be in compliance with the interests, desires, and talents of the individual?

Care givers would need to answer the following with respect to the association between prevention of hazards and promotion of normal human functioning and development:

1 What hazards to human life, functioning, and development exist in the individual's environment?
2 What will happen to an individual if a hazard is not eliminated or controlled?
3 What patterns of action should individuals develop and exercise in order to become aware of or prevent or control hazards?
4 What individual interests, values, and actions with respect to known hazards are causing conditions that impair human structure and functioning or are obstacles to normal human functioning and development?

Meeting the universal self-care requisites through self-care or dependent care is an integral part of the daily living of individuals and their social groups, but it tends to become separated from the fabric of human life when certain conditions predominate. These conditions include (1) contamination of air, water, and food with noxious materials, (2) scarcity of food and water, (3) conditions that adversely affect the work, recreational, educational, and religious activities and the daily living patterns of human groups, and (4) illness, defects, specific pathology, and disability of social group members. Under such conditions individuals as well as the social group as a whole will focus attention on these self-care requisites and may act to bring about conditions under which they can be effectively met.

Each of the eight universal self-care requisites from either a qualitative (kind) or a quantitative (amount) perspective or both becomes differentiated for individuals or groups in relation to differences in age, sex, developmental state, health state, sociocultural orientation, and resources. The varieties of practice within social groups and the range of practices used by individuals reflect not only long-term adjustment to environmental conditions but also the kind and amount of knowledge that has been acquired, is transmitted, and is put to use with respect to these universal requisites for care.

Developmental Self-Care Requisites

In the first edition these requisites were subsumed under the universal self-care requirements. They have since been separated out to emphasize their importance and because of their number and diversity. Developmental self-care requisites are either specialized expressions of universal self-care requisites that have been particularized for developmental processes or they are new requisites derived from a condition (e.g., pregnancy) or associated with an event (e.g., loss of a spouse or a parent).

There are two categories of developmental self-care requisites:

1 The bringing about and maintenance of living conditions that support life processes and promote the processes of development, that is, human progress toward higher levels of the organization of human structures and toward maturation during:

    a The intrauterine stages of life and the process of birth
    b The neonatal stage of life when (1) born at term or prematurely and (2) born with normal birth weight or low birth weight
    c Infancy
    d The developmental stages of childhood, including adolescence and entry into adulthood
    e The developmental stages of adulthood
    f Pregnancy either in childhood or adulthood

2 Provision of care either to prevent the occurrence of deleterious effects of conditions that can affect human development (type 2.1) or to mitigate or overcome these effects (type 2.2) from conditions, such as:

    a Educational deprivation
    b Problems of social adaptation
    c Failures of healthy individuation
    d Loss of relatives, friends, associates
    e Loss of possessions, loss of occupational security
    f Abrupt change of residence to an unfamiliar environment
    g Status-associated problems
    h Poor health or disability
    i Oppressive living conditions
    j Terminal illness and impending death

The first category of developmental self-care requisites articulates with each of the eight universal self-care requisites. The requisites in this category when effectively met should contribute to the prevention of developmental disorders and promote development in accord with the human potential.

The types of problems named in the second category do not constitute an exhaustive list. In some nursing situations the kinds of problems named may be a central focus of care, while in other situations, the results of the problems are considered a qualification on action within the particular situation. For example, the developmental problem of "failure of healthy individuation" may provide a central, organizing focus for nursing action in some child nursing situations. On the other hand, the arrested cognitive development of an adult, associated with "educational deprivation," may be accepted as a qualification on action since it is not likely to change during the duration of a nursing situation. Nurses will move to help patients learn and develop personally regardless of their stage of cognitive development, but the methods used will be selected in light of the stage of operational knowing the patient has achieved. The following excerpt from descriptive materials about one member of an adult ambulatory population exemplifies this nursing approach.

> Mr. M. is a 66-year-old diabetic who has never been to school, who thinks very concretely, who cannot read, who can distinguish colors but not name them, and who has fairly good motor ability. Recently he was asked to begin testing his urine at home and the nurse began teaching him. Content had to be broken into small units and presented slowly. After two sessions Mr. M. did learn to test his urine and repeated demonstrations by him at subsequent clinic visits indicate that he continues to do it accurately. As a result the clinic staff can be certain that they have accurate information about test results. Mr. M. is extremely pleased at having learned to do this and views this as an important *self-development*. During his last clinic visit he said to me, "You know, I've had this diabetes 4 years now and nobody ever did as much for me till I got tied up to this nurse. She done more for me in this time and now I know more than I did before."[3]

Health-Deviation Self-Care Requisites

These self-care requisites exist for persons who are ill, are injured, have specific forms of pathology including defects and disabilities, and who are under medical diagnosis and treatment. Obvious changes in human structure (edematous extremities, tumor masses), in physical functioning (difficult breathing, limited movement of a joint), or in behavior and habits

---

[3]Joan M. Backscheider, "The Use of Self as the Essence of Clinical Supervision in Ambulatory Patient Care," *Nursing Clinics of North America*, December 1971, p. 789.

of daily living (extreme irritability in relations with others, sudden changes in mood, loss of interest in life) focus a person's attention on himself or herself. These changes may raise questions. What is wrong? Why is this happening? What should I do? Family members and friends may also ask the same questions when they observe these obvious deviations from health. Changes that occur subtly and gradually are not detected as quickly as those that appear suddenly and dramatically. In instances where inability to focus attention or attend to oneself is part of the disease process (for example, a cerebral accident), manifestations of the disease may be noted first by family members or co-workers. When a change in health state brings about total or almost total dependence on others for the needs to sustain life or well-being, the person moves from the position of *self-care agent* to that of *patient or receiver of care*. Parents also experience a similar change in position when a child's health deviation demands care that exceeds their capacities as *child care agents*. Evidence of health deviations leads to demands for determining what should be done to restore normalcy. In modern society this would be expressed as a demand for medical diagnosis and treatment. Seeking and participating in medical care for health deviations are self-care actions.

Health deviations may bring about feelings of illness, of being sick, of not being able to function normally. These feelings, which are related directly or indirectly to the nature of the health deviation, will influence what the person may choose to do. Disease processes may also be functional in individuals and may not be accompanied by feelings of illness. The localized or generalized nature of the effects of disease or injury are related to feelings of illness. For example, a person with a simple fracture may feel well despite some discomfort, but a person with a "cold" may feel quite ill. In either situation, a disease or injury is something to be lived with and lived through since disease and injury are processes which have some duration over time. The duration varies with the nature of the disease or injury. Some disease processes terminate only with death, and other diseases are brought under control by biological processes with or without human intervention using medically derived measures. The characteristics of health deviations as processes extending over time determine the kinds of care demands that individuals experience as they live with the effects of pathological or abnormal processes and live through the duration of the process.

Disease or injury affects not only specific structures and physiological or psychological mechanisms but also integrated human functioning. When integrated functioning is seriously affected (severe mental retardation, comatose states, autism), the individual's powers of agency are seriously impaired either permanently or temporarily. Conditions that limit physical mobility, even when such limitations are severe, may be less disruptive of integrated human functioning than emotional and mental disorders. Extreme limitations of physical mobility or sensory deprivation as in total blindness may lead to emotional and mental problems, which, if unresolved, can interfere with human integrated functioning. Whenever health deviations result in disfigurement or disability, there is a demand for specialized medical and nursing assistance to prevent further deviations in human functioning.

Self-care requisites arise not only from disease, injury, disfigurement, and disability but also from medical care measures prescribed or performed by physicians. Medical care measures may modify structure (surgical removal of organs) or require behavioral modification (control of fluid intake). Pain, discomfort, and frustration resulting from medical care also create requisites for self-care to bring relief. Some medical care measures introduce hazards into the person's life situation. For example, the possibility of dependence on prescribed drugs or the risks attendant upon anesthesia and major surgical intervention are real problems. The use of these measures necessitates the use of protective care measures. The specific techniques of medical diagnosis and treatment used will produce particular self-care requisites. Nurses must know and be alert to these results and requisites.

This analysis of health-deviation self-care has shown that in abnormal states of health self-care requisites arise from both the disease state and the measures used in its diagnosis or treatment. Understanding these types of self-care requisites requires a foundation of knowledge in medical science and medical technology. Modern medical advances require nurses to be well-grounded in pathology and in various medical technologies if they are to effectively assist individuals with heath-deviation self-care. If persons with health deviations are to become competent in managing a system of health-deviation self-care, they must also be able to apply relevant medical knowledge to their own care.

There are six categories of health-deviation self-care requisites:

1 Seeking and securing appropriate medical assistance in the event of exposure to specific physical or biological agents or environmental conditions associated with human pathological events and states, or when there is evidence of genetic, physiological, or psychological conditions known to produce or be associated with human pathology
2 Being aware of and attending to the effects and results of pathological conditions and states
3 Effectively carrying out medically prescribed diagnostic, therapeutic, and rehabilitative measures directed to the prevention of specific types of pathology, to the pathology itself, to the regulation of human integrated functioning, to the correction of deformities or abnormalities, or to compensation for disabilities

4 Being aware of and attending to or regulating the discomforting or deleterious effects of medical care measures performed or prescribed by the physician

5 Modifying the self-concept (and self-image) in accepting oneself as being in a particular state of health and in need of specific forms of health care

6 Learning to live with the effects of pathological conditions and states and the effects of medical diagnostic and treatment measures in a life-style that promotes continued personal development

CALCULATION OF THE THERAPEUTIC SELF-CARE DEMAND

The calculation of the therapeutic self-care demand for an individual or group involves the following operations:

1 Particularization of each universal self-care requisite and identification of and particularization of existing, emerging, or projected developmental and health-deviation self-care requisites

2 Identification of internal or external factors that will affect the way in which each self-care requisite can be met and therefore condition the selection of methods for meeting them

3 Identification of interrelationships among the universal self-care requisites, between the universal self-care requisites and the developmental and health-deviation self-care requisites, and between the developmental and health-deviation requisites

4 Determination of if and how the methods selected for meeting specific self-care requisites will affect meeting other self-care requisites

5 Design of the courses of action through which the particular universal self-care requisites will be met in relation to courses of action for meeting developmental and health-deviation requisites

6 Formulation of a total design for self-care action that is valid for a specified duration, including points of articulation with elements of the broader system of daily living

The calculation of the self-care or infant or child care demand requires antecedent knowledge of human structure and functioning, human growth and development, family life, occupational life, and preventive health care. It also requires current and historical information about particular individuals and groups. There is also a need for up-to-date information about valid and reliable processes or technologies for (1) identifying the presence and effects of factors that affect the values of self-care requisites or limit the methods that can be used for meeting requisites and (2) meeting specific care requisites. Methods for meeting self-care requisites should be examined and understood within the cultural context of social groups and within the total care systems of social group members. Some self-care or child care measures in use within social groups may be effective and therapeutic, but health care professionals who are outsiders may perceive these measures as harmful, take steps to change them, and thereby harm individual social group members.

The adult individual gradually comes to have some understanding of his or her own self-care demands through an accumulation of day-to-day experiences, and parents often come to understand the care demands of their children in this fashion. Persons who are care agents for socially dependent individuals should be able to calculate the current and projected self-care demands on those under their care. Adolescents and adults ideally develop knowledge and skills that will enable them to calculate their own self-care demands in relation to developmental processes, to events in the life cycle, and to a range of environmental conditions that affect human functioning, human development, and general well-being. The recognition of some adverse condition in the environment or in the individual or group usually results in the need to look at the totality of the self-care requisites and to identify the methods and the courses of action that will bring a therapeutic return. Nursing professionals require highly developed specialized skills in calculating the therapeutic self-care demands for persons and groups within their defined domains of nursing practice.

The therapeutic self-care demand varies according to the self-care requisites from which it is made. At least two variations occur. These are identified in relation to preventive health care.

1 A primary prevention self-care demand
    a Universal self-care requisites
    b Developmental self-care requisites (type 1 and type 2.1)
2 A secondary or tertiary prevention self-care demand
    a Health-deviation self-care requisites or developmental self-care requisites (type 2.2)
    b Universal self-care requisites
    c Developmental self-care requisites (type 1 and type 2.1)

From the perspective of preventive health care (sometimes referred to as preventive medicine), the therapeutic self-care demand sets forth the kinds of continuing health care that (all things being equal) will prevent disease or its extension, maintain health or promote a more desirable health state, and positively contribute to the individual's human development. Meeting one's therapeutic self-care demand (or that of another) is engaging in preventive health care, which includes seeking and actively participating in the care provided by health professionals.

Calculating and meeting the therapeutic self-care demands of individuals are not adequately attended to by nurses in some nursing situations. Meeting universal self-care requisites and developmental requisites is often neglected, even in institutions where patients are supposed to receive and are charged for nursing. The use of the general comprehensive theory of nursing described in Chapter 2 should be an aid to nursing students and nurses for understanding the importance of the knowledge and skills organized around the therapeutic self-care demands of patients.

The mix of types of self-care requisites in a therapeutic self-care demand indicates the complexity of individuals' continuous care requirements and is an index of the kinds of knowledge and the range of skills required on the part of persons who can act to meet the demand. Individual deficits in self-care or care of dependents may arise from the composition and complexity of the therapeutic self-care demands as well as from the health or developmental states of care recipients. Nurses need to have the diagnostic skill of identifying the self-care deficits of adult patients in meeting their current or projected therapeutic self-care demands. A related diagnostic skill is that of determining the infant or child care or dependent adult care competencies of responsible adults who seek nursing for socially dependent family members. The range of therapeutic self-care demands of individuals who can benefit from nursing (a nursing population) and the range of self-care (or dependent-care) deficits of these individuals are indications of the kind and amount of nursing required. Care demands and deficits are also indicators of the kinds of abilities that would qualify nurses for practice.

SELECTED READINGS

Brink, Pamela J., and Judith M. Saunders: "Cultural Shock: Theoretical and Applied," in Pamela J. Brink (ed.), *Transcultural Nursing: A Book of Readings,* Prentice-Hall, Englewood Cliffs, N.J., 1976, pp. 126–137.

Coggan, Donald: "On Dying and Dying Well: Extracts from the Edwin Stevens Lecture," *Journal of Medical Ethics,* vol. 3, 1977, pp. 57–60.

Feifel, H.: *The Meaning of Death,* McGraw-Hill, New York, 1959.

Fitzgerald, Thomas K. (ed.): *Nutrition and Anthropology in Action,* von Gorcum, Assen/Amsterdam, the Netherlands, 1976.

Health Hazards of the Human Environment: World Health Organization, Geneva, 1972. Especially Chapter 1, "Air," pp. 19–46; Chapter 2, "Water," pp. 47–77; Chapter 3, "Food," pp. 72–93.

Jackson, C. Wesley, Jr., and Rosemary Ellis: "Sensory Deprivation as a Field of Study," *Nursing Research,* vol. 20, January-February 1971, pp. 46–54.

Lee, Douglas H. K. (ed.): "Reactions to Environmental Agents," Section 9, *Handbook of Physiology,* American Physiological Society, Bethesda, Md., 1977.

Minckley, Barbara Blake: "A Study of Noise and Its Relationship to Patient Discomfort in the Recovery Room," *Nursing Research*, vol. 17, May-June 1968, pp. 247–250.

Peters, Ruanne, et al.: "Daily Relaxation Response Breaks in a Working Population: Effects on Self-Reported Measures of Health, Performance and Well-Being," *American Journal of Public Health*, vol. 67, October 1977, pp. 946–953.

Rabischon, Paulette: "Pica Practice and Other Hand-Mouth Behavior and Children's Developmental Level," *Nursing Research*, vol. 20, January-February 1971, pp. 4–16.

Sartwell, Philip (ed.): *Maxcy-Rosenau Preventive Medicine and Public Health*, 10th ed., Appleton-Century-Crofts, New York, 1973. Especially Chapter 13, "General Consideration of Food Elements—Section Nine: Environmental and Occupational Health"; Chapters 22–29; and Chapter 36, "Wastewater Disposal."

Wadsworth, G. R.: "Nutrition and Public Health," in W. Hobson (ed.), *The Theory and Practice of Public Health*, 4th ed., Oxford University Press, New York, 1975, pp. 157–171.

Walker, Cleopatra, and Hazel Deuble: "A Schema for Analysis of Accident Prevention Activities in Public Health Nurses' Records," *Nursing Research*, vol. 17, September-October 1968, pp. 408–414.

Yudkin, John (ed.): *Diet of Man: Needs and Wants*, Applied Science Publishers, London, 1977.

Chapter 4

Nursing as
a Helping Service

THE FUNDAMENTALS OF HELPING

Nursing requires an appropriate education and attitude for prescribing, designing, managing, and providing nursing care. Nursing is a creative effort of one human being to help another human being. The development by the nurse of the ability to "envision" valid modes of helping in relation to "results" appropriate to a patient's condition and circumstances is the first step toward development of the art. A second step is development of the attitudes, knowledge, and skills necessary to motivate patients to achieve results appropriate to the patient's condition and circumstances. Appropriate nursing education should enable the beginning nursing student to acquire and to use knowledge about (1) the art of helping, (2) methods of helping, (3) nursing situations, and (4) nursing systems. Nurses with an appropriate attitude accept themselves as helpers to patients and as responsible for nursing acts performed and for continuing development as nurses. The nurse sees the patient as a person and interacts with him or her with this view in mind in order to seek information to form a valid and reliable picture of the patient as "being in need of nursing assistance" (a nursing focus).

Nursing is a helping service. A person engaged in a helping service performs specialized functions. Although the tasks performed may be quite simple, it is complicated for one person to do something that another person cannot do, must not do, or prefers not to do. It is complicated because the need being met is a requirement of another person. The process of giving and receiving help to meet that need will be affected by the personalities and life situations of both the person requiring help and the helper. It is recognized, however, that learning to help and helping other persons is easier for some individuals than it is for others.

We soon become aware in our daily experiences that the desire to help another person does not mean that we have the ability to do so. The ability to help other persons effectively must be developed in relation to the circumstances of daily life. Because nurses present themselves to the public as qualified and able to serve society in a special way, they must understand the characteristics of helping services as a preliminary step in becoming qualified to design and give nursing care.

Learning to Help Others

An individual may be reluctant to accept help from another person if the position, manner, and abilities of the person offering help do not inspire confidence that he or she is a qualified and able helper. As a general rule, the person in need of help will not accept help if he or she does not believe that the helper has the "right" to give help, has sufficient knowledge and ability to help, is aware of the requirements of the situation, and will act prudently. In the occupation of nursing, the official state board requirements for nursing registration and license to practice are designed to establish an individual's qualifications for rendering nursing care. Additionally, a nurse must also gain the confidence of others by demonstrating nursing knowledge and skill.

Daily we find ourselves in situations in which we are called upon to help others. Neighbors become ill and we take them to the doctor's office. Strangers ask for directions and we try to help them. These particular situations do not require specialized education, but other situations do require specific preparation for service as helpers. Nurses, physicians, lawyers, and social workers are educated so that they will be skillfully prepared to help others. Training in first aid and home nursing are other examples of preparation for helping in special types of situations. All types of helping situations have some similarities, and consideration of these similarities will be of value in learning the helping role of nurses.

Characteristics of Helping Situations

All helping situations have similar general designs or patterns. The design is engendered by the roles of the persons involved—a person who requires assistance and a person who is to give assistance—and by the expected behaviors (roles) of these persons. Ideally, the behavior of the person requiring help is complemented by the behavior of the helper. Consider the following situation:

> Two men have been in an accident. Their car skidded and crashed into a tree. One of the men, the owner and driver of the car, has suffered an injury to his back and hip. He cannot move without severe pain, and he realizes that he can prevent further injury by not moving. His companion, though shaken, is on his feet. He asks about his friend's condition and, recognizing his friend's injured state, extends assurance that help will come. He knows that he should not move his friend, so he stops a passing motorist and asks him to report the accident and request help in the next town. The motorist agrees; soon the police and an ambulance arrive, and the injured man is carefully moved onto a stretcher and taken to the local hospital. The uninjured man, with his friend's approval, arranges through the resident physician for medical care and attends to the details of the admission. He calls the injured man's family, arranges for the removal of the wrecked car, notifies the insurance company, and confers with the police officers.

In this hypothetical situation, the behavior of the uninjured man complemented the role of his injured friend. The man with the helping role communicated with a variety of persons on behalf of his friend. His communications with the passing motorist and with the ambulance attendants, physician, nurses, hospital admitting personnel, garage attendants, insurance agent, and his friend's family contributed to meeting the needs of his friend.

Further examination of the helping activities of the injured man's companion shows that the activities were directed toward achieving four goals: (1) preventing further injury to his friend, (2) securing health services for his friend, (3) taking care of his friend's property—the car—and (4) attending to his friend's personal affairs—notifying his friend's family and insurance company of the accident. To achieve these goals, the companion had to demonstrate his awareness of his friend's injured state, of the need for immobility and medical attention, and of the legal, financial, and family implications of the accident.

In this example of a helping situation, while a helper actively tried to achieve a goal or goals for another person, he had full knowledge of his actions and his own limitations. In this situation, the helper was aware that he could not give effective health care to his injured friend but could try to secure such services for him. Thus, the helper first defined and limited what he would do in relation to (1) the condition for which help was required, (2) what he knew how to do and was able to do, and (3) what was considered permissible or advisable under the circumstances.

NURSING SITUATIONS

Nursing situations have the general characteristics of helping situations. These characteristics are:

  1 There are at least two persons in the situation in different statuses, namely, the status of helper and the status of person in need of help.

  2 The status of the person in need of help is legitimized by meeting two criteria:

    a There is a need for this person to act to achieve specific purposes immediately or in the future because of prevailing conditions and circumstances.

    b There are action limitations that make immediate or future action on the part of this person impossible or imprudent or would render action ineffective or incomplete.

  3 The helper's status is legitimized by meeting two criteria:

    a The helper has identified, has knowledge of, and accepts the demand for the person in need of help to act and the person's action limitations.

    b The helper knows how to, is willing to, and does act for the welfare of the other in accordance with factors that limit what can and what should be done under prevailing conditions and circumstances.

  4 The actions of the helper

    a Complement (or substitute for) the actions of the person needing help in order to accomplish the specific purposes the person needing help should achieve

    b Provide and foster conditions to facilitate the development or exercise of this person's capabilities to take necessary actions for achieving specific purposes.

There are variations in the purposes, the requisite courses of action, and the action limitations for which persons needing help cannot immediately compensate. The general theory of nursing presented in detail in Chapter 2 provides the concepts necessary for understanding the nursing situation as one type of helping situation.

A patient with a requirement for nursing always has a twofold need for action—action to accomplish self-care and action to compensate for or to overcome an inability or limited ability to engage in care. It is the need for compensatory action or for action to help in the development or regulation of self-care abilities that is the basis for a nursing relationship. At times, nurses erroneously believe that their nursing relationship to a patient takes away the patient's rights and responsibilities for self-care or the parents' responsibilities for an ill child. A more realistic view is that the nurse provides a compensatory service or a developmental service (or both) for a patient or for the child's parents in the care of a child.

Nurses may have individuals or groups as clients or patients. Another way of saying this is to specify that the nurse's *unit of help or service* may be an individual, as in infant, child, or adult nursing situations, or a number of individuals considered together as a *unit of organization* or *a unit of service*. These multiperson-unit nursing situations include family and residence group situations. They also include work groups, schools, people in specific age groups, and people living in specific geographic locations in communities. When a multiperson unit is the patient, the individual members as well as the unit as a whole ultimately benefit from nursing.

Nurses who function at the professional level of practice have a foundation of knowledge and skills for working with both individual and multiperson nursing situations, even though they may be specialized in one or the other. The two types of nursing situations, depicted in Fig. 4-1, demand different orientations on the part of nurses because of the differences in the purposes of nurses' attention and care. In order to provide effective nursing to individuals, a nurse may need to work with some or all of the members of an individual's family and at times may need to move out into the larger community for the sake of the individual. In order to provide effective nursing in multiperson units, the nurse, though focusing on the purposes to be achieved for and by the multiperson unit, will work with individual persons within the unit and sometimes with subunits. For example, a community health nurse, who is concerned with achieving nursing purposes that will foster health maintenance and promotion for a neighborhood, will work with individuals, families, and, at times, with neighborhood groups.

It is important for nurses to differentiate between the provision of nursing to a multiperson unit and the provision of nursing to a number of individuals during the same time period. Individuals to whom a nurse provides nursing during some duration of time constitute the nurse's case load of patients or the patients assigned to a nurse for care during a time shift.

The elements of the general theory of nursing discussed in Chapter 2 were used to identify the characteristics of individual and multiperson nursing situations. The main differentiating characteristics of these two types of nursing situations are presented in Table 4-1.

HELPING METHODS

Methods of assisting have been developed and used by social group members in their efforts to help one another. The methods do not belong to any one helping occupation or profession. Parents use these methods in child care and guidance. Community leaders, teachers, and health workers

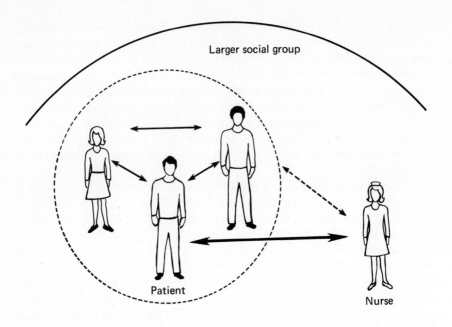

Individual type nursing situation

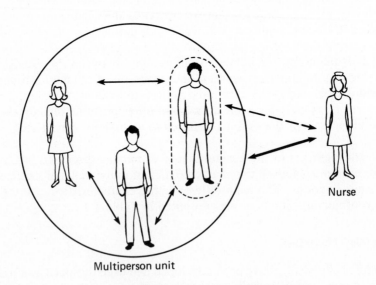

Multiperson unit type nursing situation

Figure 4-1 The object of the nurse in individual and multiperson unit nursing situations.

use them in helping both adults and children. Helping methods are also in common use in all social situations where bonds of friendship and neighborliness exist.

There are at least five general methods one person can use to give help or assistance to others. These methods are applicable in a variety of situations.

1   Acting for or doing for another
2   Guiding another
3   Supporting another (physically or psychologically)
4   Providing an environment that promotes personal development in relation to becoming able to meet present or future demands for action
5   Teaching another

In nursing a single individual in contrast to a group, all the methods of helping may be necessary for effective nursing. What self-care the patient can or cannot manage and the reasons he or she cannot manage it guide the nurse in the selection of appropriate methods of helping. For example, a nurse may decide that the judicious use of *acting for another* and *supporting another* are most appropriate for a patient who is convalescing from a debilitating illness but whose activity must be limited. The nurse would no doubt also use *guidance* and *teaching* and provide appropriate *environmental conditions*. In each specific nursing situation, one or two helping methods will probably be used more frequently than others. A change in what patients can do for themselves would require that the nurse reexamine and adjust the methods.

Specialized adaptations of the helping methods, with the development of appropriate techniques, are essential in multiperson nursing situations. The most commonly used helping methods in these situations are guiding, providing psychological support, providing an environment for personal development, and teaching. In this type of nursing situation, nurses may help family or group members develop proficiency in the use of some or all of the methods of helping. Some adaptations can be identified in the literature on health care for families and groups. Nurses must be aware of the common methods of assisting and select the methods most appropriate under the circumstances. The following discussion of the five helping methods will be useful in learning how to help others through nursing and in learning to select methods appropriate for helping individuals and groups.

Acting for or Doing for Another

Acting for another is a helping method that requires that the helper use developed abilities toward achieving specific results for persons in need of help. Examples are a nurse positioning a helpless patient, a surgeon

TABLE 4-1 Characteristics of Individual and Multiperson Nursing Situations

| | Characteristics | | |
Types of nursing situations	Therapeutic self-care demand and the self-care requisites	Action limitations and action requirements	Purposes of nursing
Individual	The therapeutic self-care demand is constituted from some mix of universal, developmental, and health-deviation requisites	All types of health-derived or health-related limitations for engagement in care	To develop or regulate the exercise of self-care or dependent-care capabilities To compensate for action limitations so that the therapeutic self-care demand will be met effectively and continuously
Multiperson unit Community groups including work group situations	There are some self-care requisites common to all persons who constitute the group Methods for meeting these self-care requisites are developed and have a known degree of effectiveness The environment in which group members work or live affects the nature of the common self-care requisites as well as the methods for meeting them	Action limitations are limitations of interest, motivation, knowledge, or skill on the part of group members There is a requirement for organized, cooperative effort to bring about the conditions and acquire resources to meet self-care requisites common to group members	To promote the development or exercise of essential self-care or dependent-care capabilities To promote habitual performance of essential measures of self-care or dependent care under known prevailing conditions To bring about the development and maintenance of cooperative efforts essential for group welfare
Family or residence group situations	The interrelatedness of members and their living environment affects the values of the self-care requisites of individual family or group members Meeting the therapeutic self-care demand of one or more individuals	Action limitations are limitations of interest motivation, knowledge, and skill on the part of group members There is a requirement for organized, cooperative effort to meet the therapeutic self-care demands of individuals within the	To promote development by family or group members of the capability to view the family or group as a unit of structure and operation To promote the development or exercise of essential self-care or dependent-care capabilities

affects if and how the therapeutic self-care demands of other members can be met

group and to promote the well-being of the group as a unit

To promote the development of the capability on the part of some or all group members to (1) plot out the interrelatedness of the therapeutic self-care demands of members, (2) design a plan for meeting individual and group needs, and (3) secure and maintain the required human effort and material resources removing a tumor from a patient's abdomen, or a mother feeding her baby. The person being helped, if conscious, must permit the helper to act for him or her. The method, therefore, cannot be used with a conscious person unless there is a measure of cooperation. Ideally, the helper assists the person in making inquiries, decisions, and plans whenever possible and prudent. The helper should also tell the person being helped what needs to be done, what to expect, and what to report. When the person to be helped is unconscious, incompetent, or unable to participate in making decisions, the helper must act with regard for the rights of the one helped and be clear about the helper's role.

The usefulness and validity of *acting for or doing for another* is determined by the type of result sought. Acting for another is not valid when results depend upon internal acts, such as control of one's own behavior. The method is valid, however, in giving care to an acutely ill person or to a physically or mentally incapacitated person according to the nature, degree, and duration of the self-care deficit. In the service professions and occupations, the method of assisting by acting for another is commonly utilized in situations where scientifically derived knowledge and highly specialized techniques are required for accomplishing a result.

Acting for another is necessary in infant and child care situations, but other methods should be added as soon as the child is ready for them. In the care of the aged or the infirm, acting for another is used in compensating for declining physical and mental abilities. Acting for another often may be gradually replaced by methods of *guiding another, supporting another*, and *teaching*.

Guiding Another

Guiding another person considered as a method of assisting is valid in situations in which persons must (1) make choices—for example, choosing one course of action in preference to another—or (2) pursue a course of action, but not without direction or supervision. This method requires that the person extending guidance and the person being guided be in communication with one another. The one being guided must be motivated and able to perform the activities required. In turn, the guidance given must be appropriate, whether in the form of suggestions, instructions, directions, or supervision. For example, a nurse may suggest to an ambulatory patient that he or she take a rest from current activity, or the nurse may discuss reasons for the limits on the patient's activities, or the nurse may tell the patient how to secure nursing assistance following discharge from a hospital. Guiding another often is used in conjunction with *supporting another*.

Supporting Another

To support another person means to "sustain in an effort" and thereby prevent the person from failing or from avoiding an unpleasant situation or decision. It also may enable the person in need of support to do something without undue stress because of the sustaining influence of the helper. Supportive activity is a valid way of assistance when a patient is faced with something unpleasant or painful. The patient must be capable of controlling and directing the action in the situation once psychological or physical support has been received. For example, a nurse may remain with and give support to a seriously ill person who is permitted to be up and to walk for a short period of time. The presence of the nurse and the nurse's words of encouragement and assurance may be needed just as much as physical help when the patient gets out of bed, maintains an erect posture, and walks. The nurse has the responsibility for judging how much the patient being helped can do or endure and when to intervene. Knowing when to step in requires wisdom and understanding. The communication between the helper and the helped (the patient) may not be in words—the helper may convey support by his or her presence, by a look or a touch, or by physical support. In other situations, speech may be necessary. A patient may need both encouragement and physical help. The action to be performed may be practicing a new skill, making a decision, or living through a stressful personal or family situation.

By giving physical and emotional support, the helper is able to encourage another person to initiate or persevere in the performance of a task, to think about a situation, or to make a decision. Support that encourages action is related to both the kind of action the person helped must take and the stressful effects of the situation. Parents, teachers, social workers, and nurses frequently use this method. Supporting another is also used extensively in child care and other situations where individuals are in the process of developmental change.

Providing another person with material resources differs from, but is closely related to, the giving of physical and psychological support. This manner of support is used by adults with dependents, by the state with respect to deprived persons, by citizens of one country for citizens of another country in greater need, and by all persons who have concern for their less fortunate neighbors. This type of support is not the specialized work of nurses. Nonetheless, nurses often assist their patients in obtaining resources from institutions or agencies. As a method of assisting, then, supportive activity may include the securing of resources. It is related to and may be a part of providing a developmental environment.

Providing a Developmental Environment

This method of assistance requires the helper to provide or help to provide environmental conditions that motivate the person being helped to establish appropriate goals and adjust behavior to achieve results specified by the goals. The needed environmental conditions may be psychosocial or physical. It is the total environment, not any single part of it, that makes it developmental. Developmental results include the forming or changing of attitudes and values, the creative use of abilities, and the adjustment of self-concept as well as physical development. Helpers may be required to provide opportunities for interaction and communication with themselves and with other persons, to give both guidance and support, and to use other ways of helping. The essence of this method is the continued and proper relating of selected environmental elements in light of the patient's special needs and the changes being sought in the patient's health state or manner of living.

Environmental conditions conducive to development provide opportunities for persons being helped to be with other persons or to become members of groups where:

1 Care is offered and provided to those with needs.
2 There are opportunities for solitude and companionship.
3 Help is available with respect to personal and group interests and concerns.
4 Individual decisions and pursuits are personal matters; there is no interference except in matters of grave consequence to the individual or others affected by the situation.
5 Respect, belief, and trust are given to others, and developmental potential is both recognized and fostered.
6 Each person expects or strives to earn respect and trust from others.
7 Each person assumes or attempts to assume responsibility for himself or herself and his or her personal development.

Physical conditions that contribute to personal growth and development provide the necessities for daily life and for psychosocial and intellectual development. For example, when an individual is tense and frightened because of the demands of daily life, *sufficient resources—* necessities as well as luxuries—*under some circumstances* may enable the person to meet particular life situations and to become better able to accept responsibilities. It must be remembered, however, that elements of the physical environment are closely related to the psychosocial environment and the social positions and roles of individuals. In assisting individuals in their development, it is not enough to supply resources. It may also be necessary to show them how to use these resources and in some instances to share them.

Providing a developmental environment is valid in many areas of living. It should be used in families, in child care institutions, in nursing homes, in schools, in hospitals, and in other organizations where human beings live or work together. The effectiveness of this method of assisting depends in large part upon the helper's creativity and his or her appreciation and knowledge of and respect for people. An environment conducive to development is also conducive to learning and is, therefore, of value if used in conjunction with teaching.

Teaching Another

Teaching another is a valid method of helping a person or a patient who needs instruction in order to develop knowledge or particular skills. Learning may not take place if the person to be taught is not in a state of readiness to learn, is unaware that he or she does not know, or is not interested in learning.

To use teaching as a method of assisting requires that the helper know thoroughly what the person to be helped needs to know. For example, a nurse cannot help a patient learn how to select foods according to a prescribed diet until the nurse knows whether the patient knows the nutritional components and caloric values of various foods. The ability to make adaptations in light of a patient's food preferences is also required. The nurse must consider the patient's background and experience, lifestyle and habits of daily living, modes of perceiving and thinking, and self-care requisites in order to be able to impart knowledge to the patient.

In teaching another, appropriate educational experiences must be provided. Teaching is not restricted to classroom activity. A nurse who is near a patient at mealtime is providing the patient with an opportunity to ask questions pertaining to diet. The nurse who explains to a patient how to perform a measure that will eventually be a self-care component (the care of a colostomy, for example) may stimulate the patient's interest in listening, observing, and asking pertinent questions about the activity. Learning to change one's behavior as it relates to self-care may require considerable time and a prolonged relationship with nurses who are able to fill a tutorial role effectively. Under some circumstances, group teaching may be an effective way of helping individual patients become efficient in self-care activities.

The interested patient may learn much from observations of competent nurses who provide care. Learning in such situations almost seems to be a matter of absorption. In other instances, a patient must engage in specific and planned learning experiences, such as reading and discussion. The learning experiences may also be related to solving problems, such as how much bread, potatoes, or rice will supply a specific amount of carbohydrate in a diet. In a self-care situation a patient may need to recognize certain effects of a prescribed medication, how to adjust the dosage, or when to call the nurse or physician. Frequently patients in self-care situations must learn to limit their physical activities. Not infrequently, patients must acquire psychomotor skills in applying supportive bandages to an extremity, skill in changing dressings, or skill in measuring and administering medication by injection.

When teaching is the helping method being used, the persons being taught ideally see themselves as learners and realize that study, learning exercises, observation of others, and practice are needed. Helpers see themselves as teachers who direct and guide learning activities. Since children and adults approach learning differently, assisting through teaching must be adapted to age as well as to past education and experience.

SELF-CARE AS ACTION

Characteristics of Deliberate Action

Self-care and care of dependents are forms of human activity referred to as *deliberate action*. This means that it is purposive goal- or result-seeking activity. It also implies that the meaning of the result sought is identified before the action is taken. This can be done at various levels of understanding. For example, adults tend to care for themselves and their dependents to sustain, protect, and promote human functioning. If adults approach care with a background of scientific knowledge, they may see results in terms of integrated functioning, as in bringing about a new metabolic balance through the controlled intake of nutrients. A person may also formulate results in terms of what he or she hopes or expects to experience, for example, to feel better or, as related to dental hygiene, to have a "fresh" mouth or, when under dental care for a pathological condition of the gums, to stop bleeding. Deliberate action is essentially action to achieve a foreseen result that is preceded by investigation, reflection, and judgment to appraise the situation and by a thoughtful, deliberate choice of what should be done. An adequate concept of deliberate action includes ideas to describe circumstances leading to the decision regarding what should be done and events and circumstances necessary to bring about the result selected. Action is deliberate when it is based on an informed judgment about the outcome(s) being sought from acting in a particular way.

Deliberate action is distinguished from physiologically and psychologically "programmed mechanisms" for responding to internal and external conditions. These are reflex activity (sneezing), instinctual urge (impulse to seek food), emotional reaction (sudden arousal of fear and movement to avoid a falling object), and feelings of pleasantness and unpleasantness (discomfort and the desire to change position after sitting for a long time). These activity patterns, however, often serve as forces motivating individuals to focus attention on present conditions and reflect upon their meaning, consider the possible outcomes of various courses of action, formulate a judgment on the appropriate action, and then decide to take a concrete course of action. This can be illustrated by an analysis of the common example of individuals deliberately maintaining specific positions for medical or dental examinations or treatments despite discomfort or even pain. Knowledge of the results of moving and not moving affect the individual's decision to control position. Physiological or psychological mechanisms and habits will affect how long individuals can exert control over their position. Deliberate action is always self-initiated, self-directed, and controlled in regard to presenting conditions and circumstances. Human development includes learning how to take deliberate action regarding the commonly encountered conditions of human existence and daily living within specific environments.

The structural elements of concrete action systems, including self-care, dependent care, and nursing systems, are discrete, that is, single actions. A discrete action (e.g., the lifting of one's hand) when taken out of its position within a sequence of actions (e.g., drinking a glass of water) may not convey the purpose and hence the meaning of the action within the particular sequence. Talcott Parsons used the term "unit act"[1] to refer to the smallest assembly of goal-oriented actions that make sense (i.e., convey meaning within a system of action). It is important for nurses to understand action sequences in terms of the discrete actions and unit acts from which they are constituted. For example, what kind and number of discrete actions must be performed to meet the self-care requisite "to maintain a sufficient intake of water" by taking the quantity of water by mouth that satisfies the criterion measures for being sufficient? Some examples of discrete actions include grasping a glass, holding a glass, and lifting a glass containing a known quantity of fluid.

Two examples of nurses' use of their understanding of action sequences required for meeting self-care requisites are given in articles by Backscheider[2] and Pridham.[3] Backscheider was concerned with the assessment of the self-care abilities of members of an adult, ambulatory nursing population to meet their particularized self-care requisites associated with the condition diabetes mellitus. To develop a standard against which to assess the action abilities of patients Backscheider analyzed the action sequences involved in meeting care requisites common to the population. Pridham investigated the same nursing questions from a somewhat

[1]Talcott Parsons, *The Structure of Social Action*, McGraw-Hill, New York, 1937, pp. 44–45.

[2]Joan E. Backscheider, "Self-Care Requirements, Self-Care Capabilities, and Nursing Systems in a Diabetic Nurse Management Clinic," *American Journal of Public Health*, vol. 64, 1974, pp. 1138–1146.

[3]Karen F. Pridham, "Instruction of a School-Age Child with Chronic Illness for Increased Self-Care, Using Diabetes Mellitus as an Example," *International Journal of Nursing Studies*, vol. 8, 1971, pp. 237–246.

different perspective. Her concern was to explore and collect data as a basis for judging the self-care capabilities evidenced by a hospitalized child with diabetes mellitus who was under nursing care. The question to be answered was: what role can the child fulfill in her own self-care? Manifestation of and criterion measures for judging the psychological development of the child (and factors affecting it) in relation to her self-care role were one focus of the investigation. Both of these investigations clearly point to the relationship between the (1) *demand* on individuals to consistently and effectively perform particular self-care actions in some sequence, with proper adjustments to prevailing internal and external conditions, and (2) their self-care *action capabilities* at particular times in the life cycle under particular living circumstances.

Self-Care as Learned Behavior

Ways of determining and meeting one's self-care needs are not inborn. Broadly speaking, the activities of self-care are learned according to the beliefs, habits, and practices that characterize the cultural way of life of the group to which the individual belongs. In some cultures, a sick person assumes that he or she has displeased the spirit of a dead ancestor and will ask a shaman (a medicine man) for help in appeasing the spirit. In a scientifically advanced culture, people assume that sickness has some natural explanation, such as an infection, an indiscretion in eating or drinking, or the presence of a growth or tumor, and they will seek care from medical doctors. Keeping the body clean is a meaningless gesture in some cultures but an acceptable precaution in others. Even within scientifically advanced cultures some groups of people may know more about health matters than do other groups in the same society. In the more knowledgeable groups, care may be taken to meet nutritional and sanitary requirements when preparing food and to secure immunization and routine health checkups. In less knowledgeable groups, these precautions may be regarded indifferently or rejected.

The individual first learns of cultural standards within the family. Hence, there are many variations in self-care practices. The child learns from parents or guardians, who learned from their parents or guardians. While growing up, the child learns of additional and improved ways of self-care from other persons: teachers, classmates, neighbors, friends, and playmates. When health knowledge is widespread and applied, the preventive care measures that are carried out on a community basis—water purification, sewage disposal, and regulated practices in the processing of milk and other perishable foods—provide not only community service but also education and guidance on a broader community health basis. Individuals in each community must provide the leadership, the daily effort, and the financial and other resources required to start and maintain these services. If there is a breakdown in community services or if services are not provided, the burden of carrying out healthful practices falls upon individuals. For example, they may be required to boil or chlorinate water after a flood or engage in these practices routinely in areas where the water supply is not safe for internal use. Some environmental hazards, such as air pollution in large cities, are relatively uncontrolled, and persons living in such areas can do little to protect themselves except by stimulating community action, remaining indoors, or changing residence.

As indicated previously, self-care requires both learning and use of knowledge as well as enduring motivation and skill. The learning process includes the individual's gradual development of a repertoire of self-care practices and related skills. Ideally, children are helped to develop images of themselves as responsible self-care agents by gradually learning to perform care measures through which self-care requisites are met, for example, bathing, brushing teeth, looking to ensure that it is safe to cross a street, not touching hot objects. Self-care measures executed daily tend to become integrated into the fabric of daily living, and the purposes to be achieved through use of the measures (the self-care requisites being met) may not be kept in mind. Openness to oneself and to one's environment and to known and validated self-care requisites and cultural self-care practices are prerequisites for learning as well as for engaging in continuous and effective self-care.

General Factors Affecting Performance

The individualized factors of age, developmental state, and health generally determine the scope of self-care activities a person can perform. In addition, each adult's established pattern of responding to external and internal stimuli will affect decisions and other actions relative to self-care. Adult values and goals also affect the selection and performance of self-care actions in health or in illness. Self-care measures compatible with a person's goals and values are likely to be seen as beneficial. Their practice, however, is dependent on the person's judgment of whether he or she can perform the measures. The first step in the practice of self-care is answering these questions: Is it beneficial for me? Can I do it? Among adults, accepting oneself as being in particular functional and developmental states and having specific structural characteristics is another prerequisite for engaging in self-care that regulates human functional and developmental processes.

THE PROVIDER OF SELF-CARE
Directional Orientations of Self-Care Actions

Learning to engage in and continuous engagement in self-care are human functions. The central requisites for self-care are learning and the use of knowledge in performing externally or internally oriented sequences of self-care actions. The *self-care agent,* the provider of self-care, is open to cultural elements in the nature of known self-care requisites and ways of meeting them. Some of these elements would be known requisites and measures of care that have been integrated into the general culture. Others would be elements that are medically prescribed for individuals or groups. *Medical* is used here in the sense of those systems of medicine that prevail within particular cultures and social groups.

The self-care provider or agent performs actions that have either an *internal orientation* or an *external orientation.* Whether a self-care action is internal or external in orientation can be determined by observation, by eliciting subjective data from the self-care agent, or both. The internally and externally oriented self-care actions listed here provide a general index of the validity of the helping methods. The four types of externally oriented self-care actions include the following: (1) knowledge-seeking action sequences, (2) assistance- and resource-seeking action sequences, (3) expressive interpersonal actions, and (4) action sequences to control external factors. The two types of internally oriented self-care actions include the following: (1) resource-using action sequences to control internal factors and (2) action sequences to control oneself (thoughts, feelings, orientation) and thereby regulate internal factors or one's external orientations (see Fig. 4-2).

Understanding self-care as deliberate action with internal and external orientations is important for nurses. This understanding aids nurses in acquiring, developing, and perfecting skills needed for (1) securing valid and reliable information to describe the self-care systems of individuals, (2) analyzing information descriptive of self-care and dependent-care systems, and (3) making judgments about how individuals can and should be helped with respect to performing the self-care operations from which a therapeutic self-care demand is constituted. When the courses of action, or action sequences, of a therapeutic self-care demand are known, they can be identified and grouped according to their internal and external orientations.

Nurses must understand self-care actions classified according to their internal or external orientations with respect to their relationships to each of the five ways of helping. For example, the helping method of *doing for or acting for another* does not correlate with self-care actions directed to the control of thoughts, feelings, and orientations. On the other hand the method does correlate with self-care actions in which resources are sought or used in controlling external or internal factors.

Self-Care and Daily Living—Two Views

On occasion, an individual must make a choice between self-care values and other values. A person who works in a hazardous occupation or

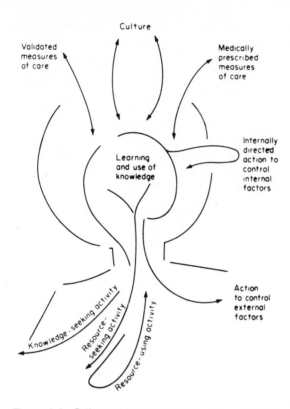

Figure 4-2 Self-care has internal and external orientations.

environment in which the risk of injury or disease is great gives less consideration to health and well-being than to other needs or desires that can be fulfilled through the job. Similarly, the mother who stays up all night with her sick child or parents who give up needed relaxation because of a family crisis are other examples of choices involving self-care.

Self-care on a day-to-day basis is interspersed among other kinds of activities or it is an aspect of another activity, for example, lifting or carrying a heavy object in a manner that prevents back injury or muscle strain. When persons are well, self-care is not a major concern; interests and activities are centered around work, special interests, and family. This is illustrated by an actual accounting for two weeks of the activities of a married woman with four children. Self-care and developmental activities are not described, nor are social interchanges with her husband and children except as these relate to her family responsibilities.

> *Housekeeping and homemaking:* taking blinds to the repairman, buying curtains, preparing meals, arranging meals so that the family could eat together.

Management of finances: balancing bank statement, paying bills, checking newspapers for food sales.

Child care and guidance—eight-year-old daughter at home: supervising child's activities as related to bathing and care of room; making dental appointment for child; helping child and friend cross a busy street; collaborating with child in making decisions about social activities; encouraging child in relation to taking a swimming lesson that day and observing child's progress at the pool; comforting child after argument with her friend; accepting, encouraging, and supervising child as she voluntarily participated in preparations for lunch and dinner; supervising child in caring for her brother's baby and communicating by telephone with her sister-in-law about the baby's well-being; supporting child as she wrote and mailed a letter to her ten-year-old sister at school.

Child care and guidance—ten-year-old daughter at school: sent cookies to child; wrote the headmaster at the school regarding the progress of the child and asked for advice for herself and husband about participation in child's remedial education program.

Guidance of adolescent—fifteen-year-old daughter at home: being available; permitting daughter to plan and pursue activities of her own selection; accepting her homemaking contributions and complimenting her on her performance of homemaking activities; in collaboration with husband, setting limits on privileges outside the home situation.

Assistance to young adult family members living in their own home— son and daughter-in-law with two babies, one of whom was hospitalized: visiting the sick, hospitalized infant; supporting the daughter-in-law, who was with the infant; discussing with the pediatrician the ill infant's problem in relation to the anxieties and concerns of the infant's parents; interpreting the pediatrician's orders to son and daughter-in-law; securing prescribed formula for sick infant from drugstore in preparation for infant's discharge from hospital; caring for the older grandchild; having son and daughter-in-law for dinner and as overnight guests.

Relations with extended family members: telephoning mother-in-law to wish her a happy birthday; talking with sister; writing to mother.

Community activities: officiating at swimming meet at neighborhood pool.

Reflection on these activities suggests how much physical and mental energy would be released and consumed. This example illustrates that time available for and needs for self-care are related to both family position and roles and to the objective situations of family members at a particular time.

Self-care is affected not only by the individual's family position and roles but also by health state. During illness, usual activities, even usual self-care activities, are disrupted and new self-care requirements may take over a large portion of a day. This is illustrated in the following self-analysis and personally recorded experiences and activities of a nurse practitioner and teacher during an attack of influenza. The recordings begin on the third day of the illness.

Saturday: Felt miserable. I knew I should see a doctor but had no energy or desire to get myself there. The thought of going seemed too much to face. Also, since I know no physician and since it is Saturday, I know I don't have the energy to hunt for one. Consulted with Joyce, a neighbor. What I was really asking was for her to motivate me to do something since I knew I would not be able to do it alone. She looked up some names and suggested that I call from her apartment.

Called the first man who handled it by telephone. He told me to treat it symptomatically (which was what I had been doing) since it is unresponsive to antibiotics. I have taken aspirin for elevated temperature, cough medicine, and hot drinks and fluids.

Up until today I felt the need to sleep a lot. Today I am not so drowsy, but my attention span is short and I have to find ways to divert myself— frequent changes of reading material, light reading only, a little knitting.

Sunday: More energy today in spurts. Felt a need to be more active with different types of things, so I repotted plants and wrapped a package. I find myself annoyed because I can't read heavier things. I keep trying, but this just increases my frustration. Read the papers thoroughly. The *Times'* cross-word puzzle is good intellectual stimulus because you can put it down and pick it up and you don't have to remember anything.

Slightly nauseated today, probably from coughing. Have to watch the "quality" of fluids. Can take juices and coke but not milk and coffee.

I am much more croupy this evening. Chest is congested. Had difficulty bringing up anything at first. In desperation I asked Joyce, who was going to the pharmacy, to bring me some tincture of benzoin [for a croup kettle]. It is good to have someone like Joyce. It makes this all seem more manageable.

Did a lot of paroxysmal coughing but finally began to cough up mucus. It is a somewhat frightening sensation. My initial reaction was to stop the coughing and not expectorate. But after doing that two or three times, I knew I had to bring it up. It's hard to do this effectively without too much distress.

Very irritable.

Monday: Soon after I got up, I took a check on the status of my symptoms. I felt better. My temperature was 98° for the first time since Thursday. I still did some paroxysmal coughing. I thought my chest felt clearer. My throat was still sore, and my ears were very stuffy. On the whole I felt I was somewhat better. I talked to two people on the phone (in process of cancelling my appointments for the day), both of whom were horrified at how I sounded. This was a shock to me since I decided that on the whole there was improvement. I realized that I could not determine whether I was objectively "still bad," but I would have to trust my own assessment of improvement.

I talked to two other persons (for the same reason), both of whom had recently had flu. Both communicated anxiety by relating my symptoms to their condition. One identified with the ear stuffiness, which in her case developed into otitis media. She suggested use of hot mineral oil drops. The other person said that it was urgent to drink two gallons of fluids a day, which I knew I could not do. After talking to each one, I had a very temporary reaction of feeling overwhelmed, of feeling aware of the importance of what each had said, but of being uncertain about it. I decided to try to increase my fluid intake somewhat and to observe the ear symptoms more closely.

I think my reaction to these contacts was to have my level of anxiety raised. On my own I had to devise a means of adapting and observing. If I had not been able to do this, I would have been left in a rather uncomfortable state.

My attention span is not much better today. I start but don't complete things. I need to be physically active but have limited energy.

My day has been characterized by intermittent naps and more frequent paroxysms of productive coughing. I continue to produce mucous plugs but feel better, and my chest feels clearer in between coughing spells.

One thing that is interesting is that with all this inactivity I have had no indication of muscle spasm in my back [due to muscle damage resulting from surgery]. I have only done my exercises twice since becoming ill [a set of exercises prescribed by the orthopedist]. On the recent trip to Georgia where I sat all day for two days, I very much felt the need for exercise. The level of my resistance to having to sit and to that experience may have made the exercise need greater. Sometimes at night after a long stretch of sleeping I awake with a feeling of being cramped, but my current need for physical and mental inactivity seems to override my need for physical movement. Friday I could not have done the exercises; today it felt good to do them. They were just enough.

Tuesday: Decided not to go to work today. My symptoms are gradually subsiding, and I would like to keep it that way. My energy comes in spurts, and I decided not to expend it in one long flame. I still have a stuffy ear, chest congestion, and paroxysmal coughing. I am losing creativity in dealing with them. They just exist now. My menstrual period began today, and I always have a little less energy the first day.

Eating is difficult, or more accurately, planning meals to eat. I just can't get interested in it. I have no idea how well-balanced my meals are. I eat if I become interested in food. I have taken too much prune juice. I have a minor gastric disturbance and some diarrhea. I have no juice on hand except prune.

I decided to walk to the grocery store, which is one-half block away. I needed to do this to test how much strength had returned. I walked there and back with my groceries and then took a nap for an hour. I am glad I decided to stay home today.

I have begun to do some work—thinking-type. I organized the class I have to present tomorrow and am writing a report of interactions with a patient I have been seeing for four months on an outpatient basis. I feel good about getting the report written; the longer I avoided it, the longer it got. It is interesting and a good stimulation but I must stop now and go sit in a chair where I can lean back and rest.

As the nurse describes her experiences, self-care was the central focus of her daily living. Adjustment of other activities to available energy was in itself self-care action. Seeking medical care was an attempt to have a medically prescribed course of action to follow in the management of the symptoms of influenza. The nurse was able to manage her own care, but not without anxiety. Some help from her friend was sought and received with gratitude. Unsolicited advice was perceived as relevant to a degree but also anxiety-producing. The difference in the objective and subjective assessments of "how sick" she was gives insight into the importance of understanding any illness as a continuum and of the need to look for change and evaluate change over time. The statement on Tuesday, the sixth day of the illness, that the symptoms "just exist now" may be evidence of human adaptation to existing conditions and the human tendency to accept and live with a situation once its novelty is lost or when there is a decrease in the intensity of stimuli.

PHASES OF SELF-CARE

Deliberate action proceeds step by step toward the achievement of some state that differs in one or more respects from the situation that existed when action was begun. Self-care or any other form of deliberate action can be described as having phases, as illustrated in Fig. 4-3. Sometimes these phases are identified in terms of managerial and productive operations, as in the sequence (1) planning, (2) doing, (3) checking—an aspect of controlling. A more comprehensive and utilitarian approach to the phases of action identifies them in terms of the kinds of operations performed and the kinds of results achieved. Deliberate action, including self-care, can be described as having two phases: (1) operations preceding and leading up to decisions about what is to be done and for what purpose and (2) operations subsequent to these decisions for engaging in a selected course(s) of action. There are other ways of describing phases of action, but this is the simplest one; other descriptions can be converted to it.[4] The operations associated with the phases of deliberate action when made specific for self-care have utility for nurses and self-care agents. The operations are indexes of the kinds of capabilities required for self-care

[4]Nursing Development Conference Group, *Concept Formalization in Nursing: Process and Product*, Little, Brown, Boston, 1979. See Chapter 7, where self-care operations are classified as estimative, transitional, and productive. Transitional operations include judgment and decision-making operations that move the self-care agent from the estimative to the productive phase of self-care.

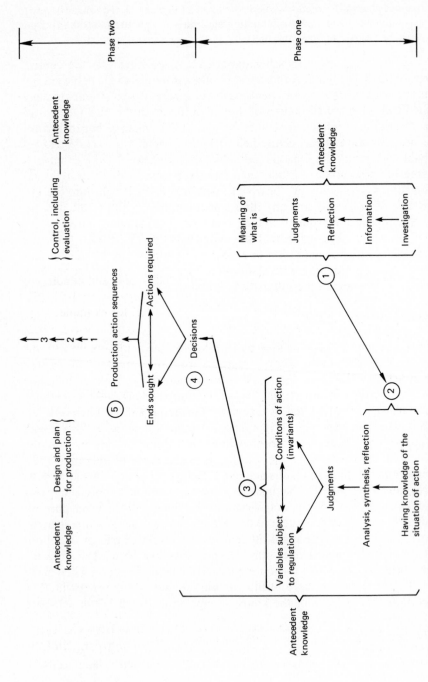

Figure 4-3 Phases of deliberate action showing operations, results, and requirements for types of antecedent knowledge.

and as such provide a basis for the description and classification of self-care limitations. Individuals' action capabilities and their action limitations, must be understood by nurses if they are to understand the nature and meaning of self-care deficits.

Phase One: Self-Care

Persons who can produce effective self-care have knowledge of themselves and of environmental conditions. They also have affirmed the appropriate thing to do under the circumstances. Before they could affirm the appropriate thing to do, they had to gain antecedent knowledge of the courses of action open to them and of the effectiveness and desirability of these courses of action. Effective producers of self-care bring the first phase of self-care to closure by making a decision about the actions they will take and those they will avoid.

Providers of self-care require two kinds of knowledge: empirical knowledge of events and of internal and external conditions and antecedent knowledge that aids them in making observations, attaching meaning to their observations, and correlating the meaning of events and conditions with possible courses of action. Knowledge extends to (1) internal or external conditions relevant to health and well-being, for example, stiffness and pain in the joints of the hands or feet; (2) characteristics of the conditions, for example, the degree of stiffness related to the mobility of the joints or the degree of the constancy and severity of the pain; (3) the meaning of these conditions for health and well-being, for example, that the identified conditions indicate an improvement or worsening of a diagnosed joint disorder; and (4) the beneficial or harmful results that will come about by taking one course of action in preference to another, for example, consulting the physician, resuming a prescribed therapeutic regimen that has been neglected, or using the affected parts of the body. The qualitative and quantitative requirements for empirical and antecedent knowledge are related to the number and kinds of self-care requisites, methods for meeting them, external conditions, including the location and availability of resources, and other factors.

Under a daily living routine, self-care requisites follow a normal pattern from which there may be little deviation. The decisions of an adult in regard to meeting self-care requisites are "programmed" in the sense that experience A calls for deliberate action B. When a person is in ill health, however, the usual pattern of the therapeutic self-care demand changes. The ill person may experience new and more self-care requisites in a totally different time distribution, and more knowledge and effort would be needed to arrive at valid judgments about self-care. In fact, medical or nursing assistance may be necessary for the judgments to be valid.

Another self-care requisite may affect the decision making. For example, a need for food may occur at the same time that a person has received a medical order to take "no food" for some time. Making judgments and decisions about self-care must take into account time specifications and the precedence that meeting one self-care requisite takes over meeting other requisites. Environmental conditions are also relevant to making judgments and decisions about self-care. The number and nature of the inquiries the self-care provider makes about environmental conditions vary with the provider's familiarity with the surroundings. A person may be half awake yet have sufficient information to decide what he or she can and will do about being cold. In an unfamiliar place a person may decide that being cold has advantages over changing air temperature or circulation.

Individuals must have some understanding of the meaning and value of self-care to make rational and reasonable self-care judgments and decisions. Level of maturity, knowledge, life experiences, habits of thought, and health state will all affect this understanding. Knowledge of self-care measures useful in meeting self-care requisites varies with life experiences. Opportunities for learning about self-care vary with families and communities. This learning process, which is continuous throughout life, is necessary for understanding self-care and being motivated to make decisions about it and to produce it for oneself and one's dependents.

Knowledge of the purposes and meaning of self-care provides the basis for appraising and attaching value to engaging in particular courses of self-care action. Factors internal to individuals may interfere with appraisal and with judgments and decisions, for example, extreme agitation, inexperience, or level of cognitive development. External factors, such as lack of resources or extreme social pressure, also affect judgments and decisions. Nurses should understand that at times self-care decisions may be based on the meaning care activities have for significant others. For example, a person decides to follow a particular course of self-care action because it will please the family. Regardless of motive, the decision to follow a particular course of self-care action determines whether an individual will take action to meet specific self-care requisites.

Knowing what conditions are relevant to health and well-being and why they are relevant at various stages of the life cycle is essential for effective engagement in the investigative, judgment-making, and decision-making activities of the first phase of self-care action. Judgments may be *rational* in that they are preceded by thought about what conditions exist and what can be done. Judgments may not be *reasonable*, however, in that they are not in accord with the existing therapeutic self-care demand and existing circumstances relating to health and well-being. Both scientific knowledge and commonsense knowledge are essential in the first phase of self-care. The investigations and the ensuing judgments and decisions made in the first phase give expression to the culture of individuals and to their self-images as self-care agents. Some individuals are reluctant to or refuse to investigate conditions that are significant for self-care. Other individuals are willing to explore what exists and what is possible but have difficulty in making judgments about what can and should be done, while others have difficulty in making the final decision about what to do. If the first phase of self-care action does not end with a decision, phase two will not ensue.

Phase Two: Action to Accomplish Self-Care

Phase two begins with the decision as to the course of action to be followed in relation to the specific demand or set of demands for self-care. The choice of what will or will not be done terminates the first phase of deliberate action. The choice made sets the goal for phase two because it specifies what kind of action will be taken. The questions raised by the self-care agent now include: How can I proceed in relation to my choice? What must I do? What resources do I need? Do I have them? Can I perform all the actions correctly and effectively at the time when they should be performed and for as long as they need to be performed? Will other duties interfere? How will I know if I am proceeding correctly? What rules will I follow? How will I know if I am getting the results I want? Who can help me if I need help?

The accomplishment of the various kinds of universal, developmental, and health-deviation self-care requires *expenditure of effort to satisfy the demands for care* as these demands are known and understood when action begins or as it proceeds. Effort will be demanded until specific results are achieved and as frequently as the result is required or until there is evidence that the effort is not productive. Effort is not random but deliberate. It is directed by the agent toward the result desired by following some standard technique or procedure or by adjusting action to the factors in the situation that can be changed or controlled. Attention is focused on the action performed and on evidence to be used in judging if the action is correct and if the desired result is or has been achieved. Deliberate effort should cease when the self-care agent knows that the desired result has been achieved. Effort may be withheld or changed if there is evidence that the result is not being achieved or that some other result is preferable. Expenditure of effort in self-care may not be pleasurable and it may eliminate opportunities for other activities.

The essential condition for the expenditure of effort to meet self-care demands in specific situations at specific times is the ability to initiate and persevere in self-care to achieve desired results. This results from (1) having specific and requisite knowledge and skills, for example, knowing how to obtain dental care, how to make an appointment, and how to describe the problem; (2) being sufficiently motivated to initiate and continue efforts until results are achieved, for example, the desire to avoid loss of teeth may motivate a regimen of dental hygiene for months or years; (3) being committed to meeting particular demands for care to the degree that forgetting is eliminated or minimized and proper priority is afforded to measures of care, for example, thoughtful performance and a routine for performing prescribed dental care are aids in consistent care; (4) being able to execute the movements required; and (5) having energy and a sense of well-being sufficient to initiate and sustain self-care effort, for example, in severe illness or disability a person may be unable to care for teeth and gums. Being able to initiate and sustain self-care effort to achieve the desired result is related to the kinds of self-care required, to external conditions, and to internal factors that affect the ability to perform deliberate actions.

Individuals may be able to initiate and to persevere in self-care action to meet universal requirements if they follow routine practices but are unable at a particular time to change old practices or to add new practices. Becoming able may involve changing one's ideas about health and illness, developing new skills, and becoming committed to new ways of proceeding. This may be very difficult for some individuals despite their knowledge that the changes should be made. Engagement in health-deviation self-care may be more difficult since abilities are specified both by the demands for care arising from the health deviation and by the medical therapy prescribed. As previously stated, specific knowledge and skills that have a base in medical science and technology are required for health-deviation self-care. Changes in medical technology have produced sometimes complicated demands for management of self-care. For example, in some kinds of drug therapy the individual may have to divide pills, take a different dose on specified days, or follow one series of doses for five days. Development of readiness to engage in health-deviation self-care may require specialized assistance. Perseverance in self-care may require assistance in the form of support and guidance.

Having some understanding of the meaning and value of self-care is fundamental to engagement in it. Some factors affecting understanding and meaning were described under the first phase of self-care. Knowledge of self-care demands and the measures to meet them is essential. Knowledge must be applied not only in the initiation of action but also throughout the performance. Knowledge must be applied to guide the performance of specific tasks and to make the practical judgments required about what to do next. Lack of skill in task performance, failure to validate judgments, or inability to make judgments will adversely affect the accomplishment of self-care. Factors in the external environment, for example, availability of resources, may affect either the initiation or the continuance of self-care action.

Initiation of and perseverance in action to meet self-care demands demonstrate the individual's power of agency in this form of deliberate action. Any action limitation decreases powers of agency and may give rise to a need for assistance. Action limitations that are related to the individual's health state constitute the reasons why people need nursing. Kinds of limitations of the ability to engage in self-care are described in Chapter 6.

SELF-CARE AGENCY

The human ability named *self-care agency,* the ability for engaging in self-care, develops in the course of day-to-day living through the spontaneous process of learning. Its development is aided by intellectual curiosity, by instruction and supervision from others, and by experience in performing self-care measures. It has been conceptualized as a unit because of the specific practical endeavor, self-care, to which it is directed. Self-care has form and content. The form of self-care is that of deliberate action and its phases. The content derives from the purposes to which it is directed, the self-care requisites, and the courses of action that are effective in meeting them.

The ability to engage in self-care is also conceptualized as having form and content. Self-care agency is conceptualized as taking the form of a set of human abilities for deliberate action: the ability to attend to specific things (this includes the ability to exclude other things) and to understand their characteristics and the meaning of the characteristics; the ability to apprehend the need to change or regulate the things observed; the ability to acquire knowledge of appropriate courses of action for regulation; the ability to decide what to do; and the ability to act to achieve change or regulation. The content of self-care agency derives from its proper object, meeting self-care requisites, whatever those requisites are at specific moments.

Self-care agency can be examined in relation to the capacities individuals have, including their skill repertoires and the kinds of knowledge they have and use, for engaging in a range of practical endeavors. Individual abilities can be described in terms of *development, operability,* and *adequacy.* [5] The development and operability of self-care agency can be affected by genetic and constitutional factors as well as by culture, life experiences, and health state. Development and operability are identified in terms of the kinds of self-care operations individuals can consistently

[5] Nursing Development Conference Group, *Concept Formalization in Nursing: Process and Product,* 2d ed., Little, Brown, Boston, 1979, Chap. 8, Fig. 8-1.

and effectively perform. The adequacy of self-care agency is measured in terms of the relationship of the number and kinds of operations that persons can engage in and the operations required to calculate and meet an existing or projected therapeutic self-care demand. Determining the adequacy of self-care agency is essential if judgments about the presence or absence of self-care deficits are to be made.

The art of nursing includes making a comprehensive determination of the reasons why people can be helped through nursing. An important aspect of this determination is diagnosing the abilities of an individual to engage in self-care (or dependent care) now or in the future and appraising these abilities in relation to the person's therapeutic self-care demand. Unless self-care agency is accurately diagnosed, nurses have no rational basis for (1) making judgments about existing or projected self-care deficits and the reasons for their existence, (2) selecting valid and reliable methods of helping, or (3) prescribing and designing nursing systems.

Self-care is performed largely out of habit, but individuals who have not thought about their self-care role may need to be helped to look at themselves as self-care agents in order to understand the values to which their habits commit them and to appraise the adequacy of their self-care abilities. Examining one's self-care habits, appraising the benefits derived from one's self-care as practiced, recognizing needs for change, and becoming knowledgeable about new self-care requisites are important for maintaining the adequacy of the individual's self-care agency. New self-care requisites resulting from changes in internal or external conditions necessitate additional knowledge, adjustments in some types of developed skills (for example, perceptual skill), and examination of one's willingness to pursue particular courses of self-care action. Persons with specific types and values of self-care requisites are important as subjects for exploratory research about the creation, use, and effectiveness of self-care practices.

Self-care agency (or dependent-care agency) is defined by qualities ascribed to individuals. In multiperson unit nursing situations profiles of individuals' self-care abilities may need to be developed in order to provide nursing. In these situations it is also necessary for nurses to know the amount and kind of cooperation and coordination required to achieve the specified purposes of multiperson units and to determine the ability of unit members to cooperate with each other and to deliberately coordinate their actions in the interest of achieving unit purposes.

If nursing is to take place, nurses must have the abilities to view their patients as self-care and dependent-care agents and to diagnose patients' abilities for engagement in continuous and effective care. To do this nurses must be able to accept individuals, families, and groups as being in specific stages of development and particular states of health and well-being. What persons can do with respect to practical affairs (including self-care) varies with age and developmental state as well as with health state. Nurses must understand the limits of the biological features of human beings (e.g., blood vessels), but they must also strive to understand the human capacities for self-care and self-management.

SELECTED READINGS

Allport, Gordon W.: "The Psychology of Participation," *Psychological Review*, vol. 53, 1945, pp. 117–132.

————:*Personality and Social Encounter*, Beacon Press, Boston, 1960.

Arnold, Magda B.: "Patterns of Action," in *Emotion and Personality*, vol. 2: *Neurological and Physiological Aspects*, Columbia University Press, New York, 1960, Chap. 6.

Benedict, Ruth: *Patterns of Culture*, Sentry ed., Houghton Mifflin, Boston, 1934.

Brown, Esther Lucile: *The Use of the Physical and Social Environment of the General Hospital for Therapeutic Purposes*, Russell Sage Foundation, New York, 1961.

Carkhuff, Robert R.: *Helping and Human Relations: A Primer for Lay and Professional Helpers*, Holt, Rinehart and Winston, New York, 1969.

Collins, Rosella Denison: "Problem Solving a Tool for Patients, Too," *American Journal of Nursing*, vol. 68, July 1968, pp. 1483–1485.

"Columbian Student Nurses Learn to Teach," *Nursing Outlook*, vol. 16, November 1968, pp. 32–33.

Combs, Arthur W., Donald L. Avila, and William W. Purkey: *Helping Relationships: Basic Concepts for the Helping Professions*, Allyn and Bacon, Boston, 1971.

Cullin, Irene C.: "Techniques for Teaching Patients with Sensory Defects," *Nursing Clinics of North America*, vol. 5, September 1970, pp. 527–538.

Daniels, Ada M.: "Reaching Unwed Adolescent Mothers," *American Journal of Nursing*, vol. 69, February 1969, pp. 332–335.

Delehanty, Lorraine, and Vincent Stravino: "Achieving Bladder Control," *American Journal of Nursing*, vol. 70, February 1970, pp. 312–316.

Dodge, Joan S.: "Factors Related to Patients' Perceptions of Their Cognitive Needs," *Nursing Research*, vol. 18, November-December 1969, pp. 502–513.

Giffin, Kim.: "Interpersonal Trust in the Helping Professions," *American Journal of Nursing*, vol. 69, July 1969, pp. 1491–1492.

Hart, Betty, and Anne Rohweder: "Support in Nursing," *American Journal of Nursing*, vol. 59, October 1959, pp. 1398–1401.

Hays, Joyce Samhammer: "The Psychiatric Nurse as Sociotherapist," *American Journal of Nursing*, vol. 62, June 1962, pp. 64–67.

Heller, Vera: "Handicapped Patients Talk Together," *American Journal of Nursing*, vol. 70, February 1970, pp. 332–335.

Henderson, Virginia: *ICN Basic Principles of Nursing Care,* ICN (International
    Council of Nurses) House, 1960.
Hladkey, Maryjayne: "Volunteer Work with a Brain-Injured Child," *American
    Journal of Nursing,* vol. 69, October 1969, pp. 2130–2132.
Kilpatrick, Helen M.: "The Frightened Patient in the Emergency Room," *Amer-
    ican Journal of Nursing,* vol. 66, May 1966, pp. 1031–1032.
McCown, Pauline P., and Elizabeth Wurm: "Orienting the Disoriented," *Amer-
    ican Journal of Nursing,* vol. 65, April 1965, pp. 118–119.
Maier, Henry William: "The Helping Process," in *Three Theories of Child De-
    velopment,* Harper & Row, New York, 1965, pp. 207–240.
Monnig, Sister M. Gretta: *Identification and Description of Nursing Opportunities
    for Health Teaching of Patients with Gastric Surgery as a Basis for Curriculum
    Development in Nursing,* master's dissertation, School of Nursing, Catholic
    University of America, Washington, D.C., 1965.
Pattullo, Ann W., and Kathryn E. Barnard: "Teaching Menstrual Hygiene to the
    Mentally Retarded," *American Journal of Nursing,* vol. 68, December 1968,
    pp. 2572–2575.
Piskor, Barbara Kovalcin, and Sonia Paleos: "The Group Way to Banish After-
    Stroke Blues," *American Journal of Nursing,* vol. 68, July 1968, pp.
    1500–1503.
Purtilo, Ruth: *Essays for Professional Helpers: Some Psychosocial and Ethical
    Considerations,* C. B. Stock, Thorofare, N.J., 1975
van Kaam, Adrian: *The Art of Existential Counseling,* Dimension Books, Wilkes-
    Barre, Pa., 1966.
Weiler, Sister M. Cashel: "Postoperative Patients Evaluate Preoperative Instruc-
    tion," *American Journal of Nursing,* vol. 68, July 1968, pp. 1465–1467.
Wiedenbach, Ernestine: *Clinical Nursing, a Helping Art,* Springer, New York,
    1964.
Wu, Ruth: "Explaining Treatments to Young Children," *American Journal of
    Nursing,* vol. 65, July 1965, pp. 71–73.

The Ability to Nurse

THE ABILITY TO NURSE

The provision of nursing to individual men, women, and children or to multiperson units such as families requires that nurses have specialized abilities that enable them to provide care that compensates for or aids in overcoming the health-derived or health-related self-care or dependent-care deficits of others. These specialized abilities, conceptualized as a unit, have been named *nursing agency*.[1] The nursing agency of individual nurses varies with (1) the form, extent, and depth of their educational preparation for nursing, (2) their orientation to nursing practice situations, (3) their mastery of the technologies of nursing practice, and (4) their abilities to accept others, work with them, and care for them through the practice of nursing. Nursing agency is the characteristic that qualifies persons to fill the status of nurse in social groups.

[1] Nursing Development Conference Group, *Concept Formalization in Nursing: Process and Product*, 2d ed., Little, Brown, Boston, 1979, Chap. 5.

Nursing Agency

The ability to nurse is a complex, acquired ability of adults who have specialized education in the nursing disciplines, in disciplines that provide the foundations for understanding nursing, and, desirably, in the liberal arts and humanities as well. Persons who have the ability to nurse have trained themselves under supervision in performing the operations of nursing practice. Nursing agency is analogous to self-care agency in that both are abilities for specialized types of deliberate action. They differ in that nursing agency is developed and exercised for the benefit and well-being of others and self-care agency is developed and exercised for the benefit and well-being of oneself.

Nursing agency can be understood in terms of the kinds of capabilities that can produce nursing actions. The static representation of nursing agency in Fig. 5-1 includes cognitive, affective, and volitional elements as well as elements that point to the skilled performance of actions. When a nurse activates nursing agency in relation to patients, the result is a series of discrete nursing actions or operations. Thus it is possible to think of the nursing agency of individual nurses as being unactivated or activated. Activated nursing agency produces nursing operations related to the self-care agency and to the self-care requisites of others.

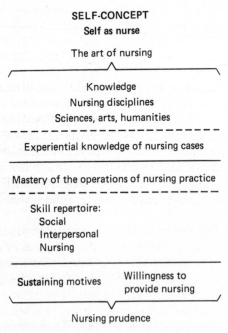

Figure 5-1 Elements of the concept nursing agency.

Art and Prudence

The art of nursing is the quality of individual nurses that allows them to make creative investigations and analyses and syntheses of the variables and conditioning factors within nursing situations in order to work toward the goal of the production of effective systems of nursing assistance for individuals or multiperson units. *Nursing prudence* is the quality of nurses that enables them (1) to seek and take counsel in new or difficult nursing situations, (2) to make correct judgments about what to do and what to avoid when particular conditions prevail or suddenly develop in nursing situations, (3) to decide to act in a particular way, and (4) to take action. Both nursing art and nursing prudence aid in and are essential for the production of effective systems of nursing assistance, but in different ways.

Through their art, nurses envision, design, and produce nursing assistance for others, assistance that is in accord with why and how persons can be helped through nursing. Art is concerned with creating systems of nursing assistance or care. Nursing prudence is concerned with doing this or that act at particular moments in light of one's knowledge of the situation. Both the art of nursing and nursing prudence develop with experience. The degree to which and the manner in which they develop in individual nurses are associated with nurses' talents, personality characteristics, developed and preferred modes of thinking, stages of personal moral development, abilities to conceptualize complex situations of action and to analyze and synthesize factual information, and the kinds of life experiences they have had, including nursing experiences.

Operations Common to the Health Professions

The ability to nurse is essentially the ability of individuals to engage effectively in one form of practical endeavor, namely, nursing, and thus the ability to nurse includes abilities of a practical and a technological nature. In the health professions where direct care and service are provided there are four general operations of practice. *Diagnosis* focuses on answering the questions What is? and Why? *Prescription* focuses on answering the question What should be? This answer is sought in relation to (1) the answers to What is? and Why? and (2) the answer to What can be? (What can be changed in the existing situation using what means?) The answer to (1) describes what exists; the answer to (2) identifies the state of the sciences and the arts with respect to changing or regulating what exists, with attention to why it exists. The answer to What should be? is also sought in relation to the known effects of action to bring about change [(2) above] in relation to prevailing conditions and circumstances. Prescriptions are made (or should be made) in light of the total situation,

not in light of some single aspect or dimension of it. *Treatment or reg-*
ulation focuses on putting into operation prescribed courses of action
(including continuing adjustment of prescribed courses of action in light
of changing conditions and circumstances). *Management of care within*
the situation focuses on the integration of diagnostic, prescriptive, and
treatment actions into a dynamic integrated system of care. Performing
these four types of operations enables one to gain factual insights (diagnoses) that precede practical insights (prescription and treatment). Management of care involves both factual insight and practical insight about
the total situation. Practical insight (following Lonergan) reveals the
"unities and relations of possible courses of action."[2]

In nursing, the performance of these four types of operations common
to the health professions has been named the nursing process. This particularization of operations to nursing requires the explicit naming of and
understanding of nursing's proper object or focus in societies. Ideally, the
proper object of nursing has become an element of a more general comprehensive theory of nursing (see Chapter 2). The listing of nursing operations in Table 5-1 demonstrates how the technological operations
common to the practice of the health professions have been made specific
to nursing practice using one general theory of nursing.

A technology is systematized information about a process or a method
for effecting some desired result through deliberate practical endeavor,
with or without the use of materials or instruments. Once a technology
has been developed and tested and information about it made available
to others, it can be further tested in practice and perfected through use
or discarded. Technologies change or should change as knowledge is
advanced through scientific endeavor. The process through which technologies are created and tested for validity and reliability is referred to
as *development*.

Specialized technologies are usually developed by members of the
health professions in relation to the purely technological work of the
profession and not in relation to the broader social and interpersonal
dimensions of work situations, but there is a need for developing and
validating technologies for the diagnosis and regulation of the social and
the interpersonal dimensions, especially in nursing (see Table 5-1). Eight
technologies used in nursing were identified in Chapter 1 of the first edition;
this list has been revised and coalesced into two categories: (1) technologies necessary for social and interpersonal (and multiperson) relations
and (2) regulatory technologies. *Social and interpersonal technologies*
include (1) communication adjusted to age and developmental state, to
health state, and to sociocultural orientation; (2) bringing about and main-

[2]Bernard J. F. Lonergan, *Insight,* Philosophical Library, New York, 1958, p. 609.

Table 5-1   Technological Orientations and Operations of Nursing Practice

1 The power of others to engage in self-care

    a Diagnose the values of the constituent elements of self-care agency of the other in terms of

        (1) Degree of development

        (2) Degree of operability

        (3) Adequacy as related to the operations required for meeting an existing or a projected self-care demand (2f below)

    b Determine the presence or absence of a deficit relationship between existing powers of self-care agency and the action demands on it (2f below)

    c Prescribe how self-care agency should be regulated

    d Represent to the other the need for and the rationale for and assist the other with

        (1) The immediate exercise of self-care agency

        (2) The withholding of the exercise of self-care agency in a prescribed manner

        (3) The adjustment or development of one or more of the constituent elements of self-care agency in a prescribed manner in order to meet existing or projected self-care requisites

2 The continuous and effective meeting of the self-care requisites of others in accordance with 1a, 1b, and 1c.

    a Diagnose existing or projected self-care requisites

    b Particularize the value(s) of each self-care requisite by determining the active conditioning effects of such factors as age, sex, developmental state, health state, sociocultural orientation, and available resources

    c Determine the method(s) through which each existing or projected self-care requisite can be met

    d Select the method(s) for meeting each self-care requisite that is both safe and effective in view of the age, developmental state, and health state

    e Set forth the courses or systems of action required to use the selected method in meeting each particularized self-care requisite

    f Calculate, in light of the foregoing, the totality of the courses of action required to meet existing and projected self-care requisites using selected methods (the therapeutic self-care demand) and then design the total action system

    g Prescribe the role that the other can safely and effectively take in self-care in light of 1a

    h Prescribe the role that the nurse (or a nonnurse) can and should take in meeting the therapeutic self-care demand of the other, including selecting and presenting valid and reliable ways of helping

    i Perform and manage role operations to meet each self-care requisite of the other according to the selected or adjusted method(s), the determined action system, and the prescribed roles (2g and 2h)

taining interpersonal, intragroup, or intergroup relations for coordination of effort; (3) bringing about and maintaining therapeutic relations in light of psychosocial modes of functioning in health and disease; and (4) giving human assistance adapted to human needs and action abilities and limitations. *Regulatory technologies* include (1) maintaining and promoting life processes, (2) regulating psychophysiological modes of functioning in health and disease, (3) promoting human growth and development, and (4) regulating position and movement in space.

These technologies (and others, including the diagnostic) are necessary for the work of the health professions and in daily life. When comprehensively developed in relation to a range of human health and disease states and to environmental conditions, they would constitute a core of technological knowledge common to a number of the health professions. Nursing and nursing education are affected by the lack of formalization of the technologies essential to nursing practice. Relevant knowledge about the processes and methods of nursing practice is widely scattered, and considerable effort needs to be expended to organize available knowledge in a form that can be applied and tested in nursing practice situations.

NURSING SYSTEMS

Nursing is action performed by nurses for the benefit of others. The actions of nurses have two orientations (within the conceptual nursing framework used in this book): (1) the ability of others to engage in self-care effectively and continuously and (2) the continuous and effective meeting of the existing self-care requisites of others in the event of health-derived or health-related self-care deficits (see Table 5-1). These orientations and the resulting organization of nurses' actions in nursing practice are described as types of *nursing systems*. The "products" nurses make for persons who can be helped through nursing can be thought about and understood as action systems made up of the actions nurses contribute with or without patient collaboration. The term *nursing system* can be used in a general way to stand for all the actions and interactions of nurses and patients in nursing practice situations. Sorting out the actions and interactions of nurses and patients leads to knowledge of the categories of action, their properties, and their organization.

A Concept of Nursing Systems

A system is anything that can be viewed as a single, whole thing. For example, self-care considered as an action system, a single entity, is constituted from the discrete self-care actions of an individual directed to meeting known self-care requisites over some duration of time. In order to understand something from a systems perspective it is necessary to uncover its structure, that is, to identify the elements that are related to each other and together make up the system and the properties of the elements. The use of a systems perspective is helpful in arriving at an understanding of complex entities.

The Nursing Development Conference Group's 1970 description of a nursing system as a tridimensional system formed from social, interpersonal, and technological subsystems is an important contribution to nursing knowledge.[3] The subsystems are viewed as interrelated but are separated analytically for purposes of understanding the complexity of nursing situations. Figure 5-2 expresses the tridimensional nature of nursing systems as a hierarchy of interlocking systems.

The concrete elements of nursing systems are the persons who occupy the status of nurse and the status of nurse's patient and the events that transpire between them. These persons are conceptualized as having attributes that legitimate their occupancy of the status of nurse and the status of nurse's patient. Legitimate patients have (1) a therapeutic self-care demand to be met, (2) self-care agency in some state of development and operability, and (3) a deficit relationship between (1) and (2), that is, self-care agency is not adequate in quality or operability for meeting the existing or projected therapeutic self-care demand because of health or health-related factors. Nurses have the attribute of nursing agency and are willing to exercise their nursing abilities for the benefit of others with health-derived or health-related self-care deficits. These attributes of patients and nurses are viewed as the variables of the technological component of nursing systems. The relationships between and among the variables in concrete nursing situations are indexes of the nature and purposes of nursing systems.

Nursing systems exist as systems of concrete action produced from the deliberate, discrete actions of nurses and patients in nursing situations. Nursing systems also exist in the form of projections that nurses (or nurses and patients) make about future actions in regulating patients' self-care agency and in meeting their therapeutic self-care demands. Projected nursing systems can exist as prescriptions, that is, statements of the type(s) of nursing system that has been judged both effective and reliable in light of the nature of and the factors associated with existing or projected patient self-care deficits. They can also exist as developed designs for nurse and patient roles and relationships that result from the selection of one or more methods of helping or assisting to be used by nurses. Nursing systems come into existence when nurses and patients operate according to their role prescriptions.

The Basic Design

The basic design of a nursing system is that of a helping system. Nursing system design delineates the structuring of the elements in nursing situ-

---

[3]Nursing Development Conference Group, *Concept Formalization in Nursing: Process and Product,* 2d ed., Little, Brown, Boston, 1979, Chap. 5.

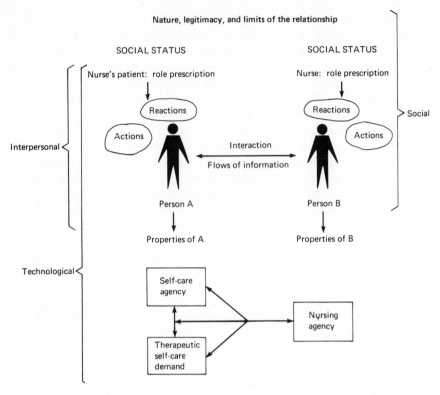

Figure 5-2 Social, interpersonal, and technological elements of nursing systems.

ations. These elements include social positions and roles, role relationships, the individuals involved, and technological elements (patient and nurse variables—see Fig. 5-2). The manner in which the elements are related reveals the structure of the system. The design of a nursing system begins when nurses select and use one or some combination of the methods of helping in nursing situations. Methods of helping prescribe general roles for the helper and the one helped. The general roles of nurses and patients defined by five methods of helping are identified in Table 5-2.

Nurses make judgments about valid methods of helping in nursing situations as they perceive factors in their patients and the patients' environments (including nurses and other persons) that are relevant to how patients can and should be helped through nursing. These judgments are made on a moment-to-moment basis, including the initial period of nurse-patient contact. Ideally, nurses see how patients should be immediately helped and foresee how they can and should be helped over some time period. The actual design of a nursing system emerges as nurses and patients interact and take action in order to calculate and meet patients' therapeutic self-care demands, to compensate for or overcome the identified action limitations of patients, and to regulate the development and exercise of patients' self-care abilities.

Projected designs for nursing systems can be developed when nurses have the necessary knowledge, foresight, imagination, and creative abilities to make a structural design for nurse and patient actions for some projected time period. Nurses who function at the professional level should be skilled in making and projecting designs for nursing systems; all nurses must have some skills in designing or in making adjustments in the design

Table 5-2   Nurse and Patient Roles in Nursing Situations as Specified by Methods of Helping

Methods of helping	Nurse role	Patient role
Doing for or acting for another	Acts in place of and for the patient	Recipient of care to meet the therapeutic self-care demand and to compensate for self-care limitations Recipient of services relevant to environmental control and resources
Guiding and directing another	Provider of factual or technological information relevant to the regulation of self-care agency or the meeting of self-care requisites	Receiver, processor, and user of information as self-care agent or as regulator of self-care agency
Providing physical support	A partner, cooperating in performing self-care actions to regulate the exercise of or the value of self-care agency by the patient	Performer of actions to meet self-care requisites or regulator of the exercise of or the value of self-care agency in cooperation with a nurse
Providing psychological support	An "understanding presence";* a listener, a person who can institute the use of other methods of helping if necessary	A person confronting, resolving, and solving difficult problems or living through difficult situations
Providing an environment that supports development	Supplier and regulator of essential environmental conditions and a significant other in a patient's environment	A person who is confronted with living and caring for himself or herself in a way and in an environment that supports and promotes personal development

*Adrian van Kaam, *The Act of Existential Counseling,* Dimension Books, Wilkes-Barre, 1966. The term "understanding presence" is from van Kaam.

Table 5-2 Nurse and Patient Roles in Nursing Situations as Specified by Methods of Helping (*Continued*)

Methods of helping	Nurse role	Patient role
Teaching	Teacher of: Knowledge describing and explaining self-care requisites and the therapeutic self-care demand Methods and courses of action to meet self-care requisites Methods of calculating the therapeutic self-care demand Methods of overcoming or compensating for self-care action limitations Methods of managing self-care	Learner, engaged in the development of knowledge and skills requisite for continuous and effective self-care

of nursing systems. Projected designs for nursing systems for patients are analogous to an architectural blueprint. Projected and emerging designs of nursing systems make clear (1) the scope of the nursing responsibility in health care situations, (2) the general and specific roles of nurses and patients, (3) reasons for nurses' relationships with patients, and (4) the kinds of actions to be performed and the performance patterns of nurses' and patients' actions in regulating patients' self-care agency and in meeting their therapeutic self-care demand.

TYPES OF NURSING SYSTEMS

On the principle that either nurses or patients or both nurses and patients can act to meet patients' self-care requisites, three basic variations in nursing systems are recognized: (1) *wholly compensatory* nursing systems, (2) *partly compensatory* nursing systems, and (3) *supportive-educative* (developmental) nursing systems.[4] This typology of nursing systems is associated with the question, Who can or should perform those self-care

[4]It should not be assumed that there is a direct correlation between these types of nursing systems and hospital patient service units referred to as critical or intensive care, intermediate care, and self-care units. In some self-care units nursing may not be provided; at most there may be some general surveillance from nurses. In intermediate care units, wholly compensatory as well as partly compensatory nursing systems may be required by patients. The same may be true in intensive care units. These patient service units are organized according to the principle of the acuteness of illness and rapidity of expected change in the condition of patients and to patients' ambulatory states.

actions (phase one or phase two actions) that require movement in space and controlled manipulation? If the answer is the nurse, the system of nursing is wholly compensatory because a nurse should be compensating for a patient's total inability for (or proscriptions against) engaging in self-care activities that require controlled ambulation and manipulative movements. If the answer is that the patient can perform some but not all self-care actions requiring controlled ambulation and manipulative movements, then the nursing system should be considered partly compensatory. If the answer is that the patient can and should perform all self-care actions requiring controlled ambulation and manipulative movements, the nursing system should be of the supportive-educative (developmental) type. Figure 5-3 provides an overview of the basic nursing systems.

These three types of nursing systems describe what would be a good organization of the actions of nurses and patients under three conditions: (1) the patient has physiological or psychological limitations for controlled movement in the accomplishment of required self-care;(2) the patient has a self-care requisite to limit energy expenditures because of health state; and (3) the patient lacks knowledge or skill or is psychologically unready to perform self-care actions requiring controlled movement that must be performed only once or performed continuously for some time but are technically complex and require informed judgments and decisions at each step of execution. The types are also paradigms of nursing systems that vary over a range. Max Black's description of range words and range definitions is a useful guide for understanding the process for identifying the three types of nursing systems as well as in identifying possible subtypes.[5]

These systems are derived from and relevant to individual type nursing situations. When multiperson units such as families are served by nurses the resulting nursing systems are usually combinations of the features of partly compensatory and supportive-educative nursing systems. It is within the realm of possibility that families or residence groups would need wholly compensatory nursing systems under some circumstances, but it is advisable at this stage of the development of nursing knowledge to confine the use of the three nursing systems to situations where individuals are the units of care or service.

Wholly Compensatory Nursing Systems

The patient factor that is the criterion measure for identifying the need for a wholly compensatory nursing system is the inability to engage in those self-care actions requiring self-directed and controlled ambulation

[5]Max Black, *Problems of Analysis: Philosophical Essays*, Ithaca, N.Y., Cornell University Press, 1954, p. 29.

98

and manipulative movement or the medical prescription to refrain from such activity (a health-deviation self-care requisite). Three subtypes of wholly compensatory nursing systems are recognized. Each subtype is based on a complex of limitations for deliberate action that interferes with

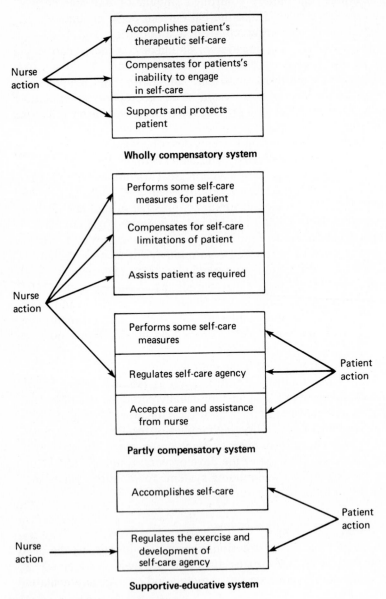

Figure 5-3 Basic nursing systems.

controlled movements necessary for deliberate actions, including self-care. Persons with these limitations are socially dependent on others for their continued existence and well-being. The subtypes are:

1 Nursing systems for persons unable to engage in any form of deliberate action, for example, persons in coma

2 Nursing systems for persons who are aware and who may be able to make observations, judgments, and decisions about self-care and other matters but cannot or should not perform actions requiring ambulation and manipulative movements

3 Nursing systems for persons unable to attend to themselves and make reasoned judgments and decisions about self-care and other matters but who can be ambulatory and may be able to perform some measures of self-care with continuous guidance and supervision

Persons who fit the first subtype of wholly compensatory nursing are (1) unable to control their position and movement in space, (2) unresponsive to stimuli or responsive to internal and external stimuli through hearing and feeling, or (3) unable to monitor the environment and convey information to others because of loss of motor ability. These persons will be confined to one location in space, unless they are moved by others. They must be protected and cared for. The valid helping method is that of doing and acting for. Nurses and others should speak to these persons using a conversational tone, handle them gently, maintain continuous or frequent contact, and maintain environmental conditions that protect and support normal functioning.

Persons whose action limitations fit the second subtype differ from persons in the first subtype by being (1) aware of themselves and their immediate environment and able to communicate with others (communication powers may be normal or greatly restricted); (2) unable to move about and perform manipulative movements because of pathological processes or the effects or results of injury, immobilizing measures of medical treatment, or extreme weakness or debility; or (3) under medical orders to restrict movement. These persons may be mentally competent and capable of making accurate observations. They may be involved in making judgments and decisions about self-care and perform self-care actions that do not require movement. They must exercise self-control and develop a style of living that promotes normalcy of outlook and continued personal development and must maintain their willingness to be cared for by others regardless of their reluctance to do so. Nurses use a number of methods of helping patients in the second subtype, with emphasis on maintaining a developmental environment and doing and acting for the patient. Patients with these limitations will suffer when neglected by nurses and others and when their interests and concerns are not solicited or are ignored. Psychological support, guidance and directon, and teaching are therefore valid methods also. Prevention of hazards and promotion of normalcy must be given special attention because of the possible deleterious effects of inactivity, restricted environments, and awareness of one's helplessness.

Persons in the third category differ from those in the first two subtypes in that (1) they are conscious but are unable to focus attention on themselves or others for purposes of self-care or care of others, (2) they do not make rational or reasonable judgments and decisions about their own care and daily living without guidance, or (3) they can ambulate and perform some measures of self-care with continuous guidance and supervision. Persons characterized by such limitations bring about hazardous conditions for themselves and, at times, for others. They should be cared for and protected, and others may need to be protected from them. The helping methods associated with this set of limitations include providing and maintaining a developmental environment, guiding and directing, providing support, and doing or acting for.

Wholly compensatory nursing systems have social and interpersonal and technological dimensions that must be understood by nurses. These dimensions are related to the extremely restricted ability or inability of persons to manage themselves and to control environmental conditions. From the nursing viewpoint, nurses are not only major providers and managers of patients' self-care, they are also the makers of judgments and decisions about the self-care requisites of their patients and the designers of nursing care. Nurses have the responsibility to meet all three types of self-care requisites—universal, developmental, and health-deviation—for persons with the types of limitations described here. Nurses must be in close contact and communication with family members, know who is responsible for the patient's affairs, and be able to sort out the nursing responsibility for the patient from family members' rights and responsibilities. The social, interpersonal, and technological dimensions of these nursing situations require that nurses be the major and, in some instances, the sole contributors to action systems produced to meet the self-care requisites of patients and protect patients' powers of self-care agency and their personal integrity.

Because of the labor involved in providing continuous care to persons with the action limitations identified here, persons other than nurses are frequently placed in positions of responsibility for patients requiring wholly compensatory nursing systems. Nurses have a social responsibility as members of the nursing profession to act to ensure safe and effective care to persons with extensive limitations of the self-care agency. This responsibility can be fulfilled when nurses are free enough as professionals to accept the responsibility and are creative and knowledgeable enough to design, put into operation, and manage effective care systems for these persons. They should also be knowledgeable enough to set the specifications for and guide and supervise others who can contribute to the operation of wholly compensatory care systems.

Partly Compensatory Systems

The second system is for situations where both nurse and patient perform care measures or other actions involving manipulative tasks or ambulation. The distribution of responsibility to nurse or patient for performance of care measures varies with (1) the patient's actual or medically prescribed limitations for ambulation and manipulative activities, (2) the scientific and technical knowledge and the skills required, or (3) the patient's psychological readiness to perform or learn to perform specific activities. The patient or the nurse may have the major role in the performance of care measures. A partly compensatory nursing system may take a number of forms. In one form, patients perform universal measures of self-care and nurses perform medically prescribed measures and some universal self-care measures. A second form is for these situations where patients are learning to perform some new care measures. In partly compensatory situations all five helping methods may be in use at the same time.

Supportive-Educative Systems

The third system is for situations where the patient is able to perform or can and should learn to perform required measures of externally or internally oriented therapeutic self-care but cannot do so without assistance. Valid helping techniques in these situations include combinations of support, guidance, provision of a developmental environment, and teaching. This is a *supportive-developmental system*. It is the only system where a patient's requirements for assistance relate to decision making, behavior control, and acquiring knowledge and skills. There are a number of variations of this system. In the first, a patient can perform care measures but needs guidance and support. Teaching is required in the second variation. In the third, providing a developmental environment is the preferred method of helping. The fourth variation is in situations where the patient is competent in self-care but requires periodic guidance that he or she is able to seek; in this variation, the nurse's role is primarily consultative.

Nursing Practice Implications

The preceding descriptions of the three types of nursing systems are constituted from the differences in the roles of nurses and patients in meeting the patients' self-care requisites. One or more of the three types may be used with a single patient. For example, patients who are receiving nursing because of surgical treatment involving anesthesia and organ removal may progress from a supportive-educative system to a partly compensatory system to a wholly compensatory system, then back to a partly compensatory system and, finally, to a supportive-educative system before being discharged from nursing. Other patients, especially those in ambulatory care services, may take part in supportive-educative nursing systems, shifting at times to partly compensatory nursing systems. Nurses should select the type of nursing system or sequential combination of nursing systems that will have optimum effect in achieving the desired regulation of patients' self-care agency and the meeting of their self-care requisites.

Through nursing, patients with extensive action limitations may develop the capabilities needed to design and manage their own self-care and to guide and direct a helper in the provision of care. With nursing consultation and medical supervision, other patients may become able to identify their self-care requisites and to design, provide, and manage their own self-care toward the regulation of the effects of pathology.[6] The descriptions of the three types of nursing systems and the criterion measures for determining the kind(s) of system(s) needed should be used in examining information about patients' self-care abilities and limitations before prescribing nurse and patient roles. They can also be used to determine whether or not nurse and patient roles in active nursing situations are in accord with patients' self-care abilities and limitations. This further development of the conceptual structure of the theory of nursing systems articulated in Chapter 2 provides nurses with knowledge that can guide their decision-making and evaluative actions in situations of nursing practice.

The utility of the basic design of nursing systems has been pointed out in relation to the specification of nurse and patient roles and the assisting techniques that the nurse would need to employ. Because of this, the three nursing systems suggested for the purposes of this text could serve as a guide in the development of a typology of nursing situations for use within health care agencies or communities. Each patient presents specific requirements for assistance that describe his or her need for one or a combination of the three nursing systems. Professional nurses are responsible for accumulating information about patients that describes commonalities and differences in their nursing requirements, including both requirements for assistance with self-care and overcoming obstacles

[6]Rita M. Sezekulla Meyer and Diana Torzeinski Morris, ''Alcoholic Cardiomyopathy: A Nursing Approach,'' *Nursing Research*, vol. 26, November-December 1977, pp. 422–427. Maria Meyer, ''Application of the Orem Self-Care Deficit Theory to Nursing Practice,'' paper given at a conference on Nursing Theories: Adaptation and Self-Care, St. Louis University Medical Center, October 25, 1978.

to self-care. The commonalities among specific types of patients, if identified in terms of factors that specify roles and requirements for specific assisting techniques, would indicate the health agency or community requirement for particular systems of nursing assistance. This information is important in planning for the number and kinds of nurses and nurses' assistants needed to provide a nursing service that will be adequate for a particular population. It is also important for nursing education.

Since the 1960s operations researchers have given attention to measuring the dependency of patients in residence care institutions on nursing staff. Methods for determining the disability status of persons living at home have also been formulated. The results of these investigations should be reviewed and brought together by nursing scholars. The conceptual constructs of self-care agency and nursing system would be useful in organizing available, validated information. Since nurses in nursing practice seek formal insights about what is and why, they require reliable methods for reaching conclusions that are comprehensive, systematic, and correct. The kind and quality of data required for making judgments and decisions about the roles of nurses and patients in health care situations should be of special concern to nurse researchers.

NURSING OPERATIONS AND NURSE CHARACTERISTICS

The title *nurse* and the title *nurse's patient* signify the social positions and roles of persons who come together with the related general purposes of providing nursing and being provided with nursing. The capability to provide nursing to others includes specialized abilities necessary for the technological operations of nursing practice and for the following social and interpersonal operations necessary for nursing practice. First, nurses need to initiate, maintain, and sever relationships with their patients and with the patients' significant others. This requires nurses to obtain information about patients, including information about personal factors such as age and personality characteristics, and to make information about themselves as nurses available to patients and patients' significant others. Second, nurses should become socialized to the nurse role and assist patients in becoming socialized to their roles within nursing situations, which are at times part of broader health care situations. Third, nurses must adjust to and help patients to adjust to changing conditions and circumstances in nursing and broader health care situations, including role changes. Fourth, nurses should cooperate with other health workers who provide care to patients by coordinating nursing actions with the actions of these workers and simultaneously helping patients to understand the points where self-care joins with other health care services needed by or being provided to them. Finally, nurses need to know the domain and boundaries of nursing and to keep their professional actions within these boundaries in order to protect the domain of nursing, as it is related to patients, from infringement by other health workers.

Nurses' social and interpersonal abilities enable them to perform these five operations, which bring about and maintain the social and interpersonal conditions necessary for nurses' properly timed and effective performance of the technological and managerial operations of nursing practice—diagnosis, prescription, regulation or treatment, and management of nursing care. Knowing when and how to engage in the social and interpersonal operations of nursing practice and how to integrate them with technological and managerial operations is a mark of the experienced nurse. Nurses who have a dynamic concept of nursing systems, viewing them as being composed of social, interpersonal, and technological elements, have a foundation for arriving at insights about themselves and their patients that are meaningful for nursing purposes. Knowing oneself and knowing the other, respecting oneself and respecting the other, and accepting oneself and accepting the other make it easier to establish cooperative relationships.

The relationships between nurses and patients vary in duration from hours to days to months to years. Nurses must be able to enter into short-term and long-term relationships with patients with a view toward rendering effective help for short periods of time or over a prolonged period of time with either periodic or continuous contact. Regardless of the duration of contact and the patient's specific nursing requirements, nurses must have the knowledge, the enduring attitudes, the willingness, and the skills necessary for helping their patients with self-care and with regulating patients' self-care agency. Desirable nurse characteristics in relation to the social, interpersonal, and technological dimensions of nursing practice necessary for the design, production, and management of effective nursing systems are suggested below.

SUGGESTED DESIRABLE NURSE CHARACTERISTICS

Social

1 Is well informed about and accepts the general social and legal dimensions of nursing situations; has specialized knowledge of the particular social and legal dimensions of some types of nursing situations

2 Has knowledge of cultural differences between social groups and among members of social groups and understands the significance of people's cultural orientations in their contacts and communications with others

3 Has a repertoire of social skills, including communication skills, sufficient for effecting and maintaining contacts with individuals and multiperson units from a range of social classes and culture groups

4 Accepts and respects himself or herself and others as developing persons, recognizing that each person has characteristic ways of conducting himself or herself in interpersonal situations

5 Is courteous and considerate of others

6 Is responsible in the provision of nursing to individuals or multiperson units within defined types of nursing situations

7 Understands the domain and boundaries of nursing as one of the health services provided for by society

8 Understands the nature of contractual and professional relationships and is able to perform the operations of nursing practice within limits set by these relationships

Interpersonal[7]

1 Is well informed about the psychosocial dimensions of human functioning

2 Has knowledge of factors that facilitate or impede interpersonal functioning

3 Has knowledge of conditions necessary for the development of helping relationships

4 Is interested in identifying and resolving human problems that interfere with satisfying relationships with others and produce emotional pain or suffering

5 Has a repertoire of interpersonal skills that can be adjusted to infants, children, and adults, including those who are ill, disabled, or debilitated. Such skills enable nurses to

  a Be an active participant in relationships with patients and their significant others

  b Be a participant observer in interpersonal relationships with patients and their significant others with the goal of identifying personality characteristics (e.g., being controlling or passive) significant in the relationship and the existence and degree of emotional suffering or emotional pain (anxiety) and physical discomfort and pain (if both are severe, they can interfere with the patient's observation of events, resulting in a lack of knowledge of the interpersonal situation and sometimes in misinterpretation of it)

  c Reduce patients' emotional pain and physical discomfort and pain by effecting conditions that increase patients' comfort and satisfaction within the nurse-patient relationship

  d Increase awareness of the interpersonal situation in terms of the desirable or undesirable factors that affect meeting patients'

[7]The identified characteristics pertain to interpersonal operations needed in all types of nursing situations. Some methods or technological approaches to meeting certain self-care requisites or to regulating self-care agency are purely interpersonal in nature; such interpersonal methods are considered as being within the technological operations of nursing practice. Mental health nursing specialists caution against the indiscriminate use of regulatory technologies that are valid for use in situations where patients have grave interpersonal problems.

therapeutic self-care demands and regulating their self-care agency

6   Is able to relate to patients and their significant others in a manner that conforms to the conventional form for human interactions (e.g., making eye contact when engaged in conversation, maintaining a conversational tone when seeking information)

7   Has a repertoire of communication skills (adjusted to the age and developmental state of individuals, their cultural practices, and communication problems resulting from genetic defects and pathological processes) sufficient for effecting and maintaining relationships essential in the production of wholly compensatory, partly compensatory, and supportive-educative nursing systems for patients

8   Accepts persons who are under nursing care and works with them in accordance with their roles in self-care and dependent care

9   Identifies broader social and legal aspects of interpersonal situations (e.g., who is legally responsible for the patient) and is able to represent these in a prudent way to patients or their significant others

Technological

1   Has mastery of valid and reliable techniques for nursing diagnosis and prescription; for meeting the therapeutic self-care demands of individuals with various mixes of universal, developmental, and health-deviation self-care requisites; and for regulating the quality and exercise of the self-care agency of individuals

2   Is experienced or becoming experienced in using valid and reliable techniques in performing the technological operations of nursing practice (see 1 above) in defined types and subtypes of nursing situations and in producing nursing systems within these situations

3   Is able to integrate the social and interpersonal dimensions of nursing practice with the technological dimensions (see 1 above) toward the production and management of effective nursing systems for individuals and multiperson units

4   Is alert, at ease, and confident in nursing situations; is relaxed but able to mobilize for immediate and effective action to protect patients' well-being and to regulate the variables of nursing systems and the relationships among them

5   Seeks nursing practice experience and supervision as well as specialized education and training to extend or deepen his or her area of nursing practice with respect to nursing populations

6   Works toward the formulation and testing of methods and techniques for technological operations of nursing practice within his or her nursing specialization

7   Strives to increase ability to apprehend those factors in nursing situations that condition the values of the patient variables, self-care agency, and therapeutic self-care demand and thus set up requirements that nursing agency be of a particular value

8 Identifies the results obtained in specific nursing situations from the use of specific methods in meeting patients' therapeutic self-care demands and in regulating their self-care agency; compiles results over time by types of nursing situations; isolates factors associated with types of results; and compares results in the different types of nursing situations

The characteristics of nurses presented above represent a further development of the nursing agency. They can be used as a foundation for exploratory studies of nurses' qualifications for nursing practice, which in turn serve as bases for research to establish the associations between nurse characteristics and the design, production, and management of nursing systems.

PERSONAL CHARACTERISTICS OF PATIENTS AND NURSES

Nursing practice situations are helping situations in which patients' self-care deficits and the nursing systems prescribed and produced by nurses result in complementary sets of behaviors on the part of nurses and patients. What nurses and patients do to meet the therapeutic self-care demands of patients and to regulate patients' self-care agency constitutes the essential core of a nursing system. It has been suggested here that this core is facilitated by (and, ideally, integrated with) nurses' effective performance of social and interpersonal operations of nursing practice. These sets of operations are regulatory in nature. They help regulate (1) the nurse-patient relationship, (2) the deliberate actions nurses and patients perform because of the deficit relationship between patients' self-care agency and their therapeutic self-care demands, and (3) human developments and functioning through actions that meet patients' self-care requisites and protect or develop self-care agency.

A question relevant to nursing practice is, What are the *limitations on* what nurses and patients can and should do in regulating patients' states of development and health in particular nursing situations? The following factors set limits on the methods that can be selected and used in meeting the self-care requisites of individuals: (1) age, (2) sex, (3) developmental state, (4) relevant life experiences, (5) health state, (6) sociocultural orientation, and (7) available resources, including time. The Nursing Development Conference Group instituted the use of the term *basic conditioning factors* to refer to these patient characteristics because of their qualifying influence on the two patient variables of nursing systems. Since these patient characteristics also limit nursing agency or its exercise, they were also recognized as being personal characteristics of nurses that can affect nursing practice.

Personal Characteristics of Patients

Gathering personal information about patients and perceiving its meaning for nursing is a nursing practice operation that contributes to nurses' performance of the social, interpersonal, and technological operations identified in this chapter; it is often made a part of the three operations. The quality of and the amount of information essential for effective nursing practice depends in this instance upon why and how individuals can be helped through nursing and the complementary roles of nurses and patient in a system of care. In initial contacts with persons who are under or who are seeking nursing care or from available records, nurses should determine:

    1 Reasons why health care, including nursing, is being sought or received

    2 Experiences of the person in similar situations

    3 Age, sex, position in family (family of origin, family of marriage), or membership in a residence group

    4 Gross evidence of developmental state by stage of the life cycle

    5 Gross evidence of health state, for example, ability to control position and movement in space; signs of injury, debility, illness; sensory impairment

    6 National origins, language, place of residence, religious orientation, and nature of occupational or educational endeavors

This information should aid nurses in managing themselves in nursing situations and should enable them to understand how these patient characteristics limit or qualify the values of the nursing system variables and the operations of nursing practice.

As nursing diagnosis proceeds, nurses obtain more detailed information (to the degree required) about developmental state, health state, conditions of living and life-style, and economic resources since these are relevant to (1) having knowledge of patients' current self-care systems; (2) determining existing and projected self-care requisites and particularizing them to existing and changing factors in patients or their environments; (3) determining the factors in patients or their environments that condition the ways in which self-care requisites can be effectively met; and (4) determining factors in patients or their environments that limit or qualify the development, operability, or adequacy of self-care agency. The personal characteristics of patients can also be used to arrive at insights about the state of individual patients. From this perspective, the seven conditioning factors listed on page 107 can be considered together as a *vector*[8] that describes, for nursing purposes, the state of a nurse's

---

[8]W. Ross Ashby, *An Introduction to Cybernetics*, Chapman & Hall, Ltd., London, 1956. See pp. 30–31, where a vector is defined as a "compound entity, having a definite number of components."

patient. The condition of the patient is described in terms of less comprehensive states, for example, in terms of age, sex, or state of anatomical,
physiological, psychological, or psychosocial development. Since states
of persons cannot be specified in terms of a single component, the personal
characteristics of patients should be considered by nurses as relevant to
what nurses and patients do in nursing situations.

Nursing Meaning of Patient Characteristics

When identified, the *sex, age, and physical, intellectual, and emotional
manifestations of growth and development* of a patient enable the nurse
to make judgments about the patient's ability to engage in purposeful self-
care activities. Judgments can also be made on the relationship of a patient's growth and development to norms for his or her age group and sex
and the adjustments in self-care requisites that will be necessary because
the patient is either below or has exceeded the norms for his or her sex
and age group.

In gathering information about the patient's *characteristic behavior*
in life situations, the nurse will want to learn how the patient perceives
and reacts in commonly experienced situations within the family or the
community, in contrast with his or her reaction to illness, to medical care,
to strangers, and to stress-producing situations such as the illness of a
spouse, the death of a close family member or friend, or failure in school
or in work. The nurse may seek this information from the patient or from
the family. The nurse will also observe patient behavior while rendering
care.

Care-related information about cultural manifestations includes what
the patient customarily does for self-care and his or her self-care behavior
in the present health situation. Such information is then examined by the
nurse in relation to the health goals and the self-care characteristics of
the patient's cultural group. Data about selected personality and cultural
characteristics, when added to data about sex, age, and physical and
emotional manifestations of growth and development, enable the nurse
to develop a relatively complete picture of the patient from a nursing care
perspective.

Past and present external demands upon the patient, when identified,
enable the nurse to round out the developing image of the patient as a
person. Facts about the adult patient's marital status, family roles, occupation, and position in the community; or the child patient's place in
the family as a sibling, his or her placement in school and relationship to
parents and other adults; and what both adult and child patients say about
their physical and social environment aid the nurse in identifying or in
making inferences about external demands upon the patient. How a patient
has coped with these demands and how he or she is likely to cope with

them in light of the present or projected future health state are questions for which both the nurse and the patient will need answers.

The patient's self-expectations within a particular physical and social environment will influence behavior. Outlook on life and on the world, self-image, and habits and reactions to the environment will also influence the patient response to environmental demands.

Health state factors are directly related to the patient's care requisites, abilities, and limitations. The factors may indicate a need for new components or adjustments in the universal components of self-care. Obtaining needed information requires a background of general knowledge about each health and disease factor. Knowledge of disease, preventive medicine, and medical diagnosis and prognosis is required. The nurse should understand, for example, that a physician's diagnosis is a judgment made on the basis of symptoms, diagnostic tests, and examinations. Sometimes it is a tentative or working diagnosis. When the patient is receiving preliminary medical care in preparation for a diagnostic medical workup, there will be no medical diagnosis. The physician may describe the patient's major complaints and other manifestations of health or disease. In cases of a routine medical checkup, the physician's efforts will be directed primarily toward describing structure and functioning through a series of tests and examinations.

The patient's attitude toward his or her own health and well-being is another important health-related aspect. Adult persons are expected to act with responsibility in matters that affect their own well-being or that of others. Responsibility is a quality that is dependent on the values an individual holds with respect to a particular field of action, for example, health care for dependents. Responsibility is exhibited by a person when, because of his or her values, he or she "inhibits or controls" immediate "specific desires, impulses, or interests" when confronted with "immediate adverse conditions" in a situation where he or she must act.[9] Some adult members of society fail to act with responsibility for their own well-being or for that of their dependents. Other adults, because of poor health, social obligations, or limited resources find it extremely difficult to fulfill their duties, although they feel responsible and want to behave in a responsible manner. Dependent children and adults who are legally recognized as incompetent to manage their own affairs cannot be held responsible for their own well-being.

Personal Characteristics of Nurses

In the following discussion, *position factors* and *personal factors* will be considered in relation to the personal and role characteristics of the nurse as a person in nursing situations. Position factors include the nurse's role

[9]Chester I. Barnard, *The Functions of the Executive,* Harvard University Press, Cambridge, Mass., 1962, pp. 260–263.

as the agent in rendering nursing care, the nurse's acceptance of the need to and the willingness to render care, the actual performance of nursing care, and the nurse's acceptance of ethical considerations in human relations. These position factors describe the characteristics of persons qualified to render care.

To be able to view himself or herself realistically as a person who renders nursing care, the nurse must have the time and preparation to give the patient care. Education and experience in nursing and the scope of responsibility for nursing the patient should influence that view. Many factors affect the willingness of the nurse to render care. Some nurses frequently specify lack of time as a result of the many demands upon them. Other nurses refer to patients as "difficult" or "easy," thereby implying the kind and degree of effort involved in rendering care. The patient's age, sex, race, culture, social status, or disease factors also have an effect on the nurse's willingness to render care. In fact, some nurses develop preferences about the types of patients for whom they are willing to render care. In the last analysis, the quality and availability of nursing care in specific nursing situations is based upon the unconditional willingness of individual nurses to render care.

Socialization in nursing situations is required because the nurse and the patient are usually strangers and they must enter into a helping relationship. The patient may need preparation in fulfilling the patient role in the nursing situation. Temperament, self-image, and pattern of living may affect the patient's ability to accept the role of patient. Further, the nurse's sex, age, culture, or socioeconomic status may facilitate or hinder the patient's performance in the patient role. Similarly, these same factors, as they relate to the patient, may have an effect on the nurse's performance of the nurse role.

The socializing process may continue throughout the period the patient requires nursing care. It is not merely an initial effort on the part of the nurse and the patient to adjust to their roles in the situation, but a continued effort to carry out their roles and to understand their relationships with other persons who are providing care in the situation. The nurse sometimes must ask: "Is the patient able to participate in his or her own health care by giving essential information to the physician or to others?" The following excerpts from recorded material about a nursing case present an example of a need for help in this direction. It is evident from these excerpts that the nurse and the patient had established an effective nurse-patient relationship and that the patient trusted the nurse. The progress made by the patient as a result of his own socializing efforts is also evident. The observations were made and recorded by Sister Gretta Monnig.[10]

[10]Sister M. Gretta Monnig, *Identification and Description of Nursing Opportunities for Health Teaching of Patients with Gastric Surgery as a Basis for Curriculum Development*

The patient was sitting in a chair when the surgeon made rounds. The doctor remarked that this was enema day. The patient said nothing about the enema but told the surgeon that he felt fine. After the surgeon had left the room, the nurse remarked that she would get the enema. The patient replied, "I do not need an enema; I had a bowel movement this morning." The nurse asked why he had not told the surgeon.

"I take a look at all those doctors and can't think of a thing to say. Do the other patients feel this way?" he asked.

The nurse replied, "Most patients think of their questions after their doctor has been in to see them. It must be hard to ask questions in front of a large group of people."

"All those people scared me. I was afraid that my questions would sound silly," replied the patient.

The nurse asked, "Is it easier to talk to the doctor when he makes rounds to change your dressings?"

"He always seems to be in a hurry," replied the patient.

"How about the doctor who comes in the evening?" asked the nurse.

"He is a fine doctor," said the patient. "I usually save my questions for him, but I still forget to ask him."

"Would writing the questions on a slip of paper help you to remember what you want to ask the doctor?" asked the nurse.

"I will try that," replied the patient.

In the evening the patient said, "I wrote down my questions today. The doctor answered every one of them. He talked to me quite a while. I never realized how interesting doctors are." After that evening the patient appeared more at ease when the doctors made rounds.

Ideally, then, the socializing efforts of nurses help them to know their patients and how to direct their efforts in encouraging patients to better cope with socializing activities in health situations. When children are involved, their developmental state and physical dependence upon adults are of prime importance in the socializing aspects of the nursing situation. The nurse who gives care to children has a dual function in socialization activities. The nurse must continue, along with the parents, to aid the child in normal development. Under the conditions imposed by illness or special health needs, a child is confronted by physicians and other adults who place a variety of demands upon both the child and the parents. Fostering the child's movement toward independence during illness through socializing activities is an important nursing task. Supervised contacts with other children may be of great importance in the socialization of children in institutional settings. Some three-year-old children, for example, can effectively demonstrate to another child how to behave

in Nursing, master's dissertation, School of Nursing, Catholic University of America, Washington, D.C., 1965, pp. 89–90.

under conditions new to them—where and when to wash the face and hands, where to eat, and the proper use of utensils.

Closely related to socialization is the nurse's and the patient's awareness of overt and covert problems in health care situations. The case material on the socialization of the patient demonstrated that the patient was aware of his inability to communicate with the physicians attending him and recognized his need to change that behavior. It was up to the nurse to assist him in changing. The nurse cannot do this effectively unless he or she understands and accepts the nurse's and the patient's role in the nursing situation.

Personal factors that help to describe the nurse include (1) *age, sex, race, and physical and constitutional characteristics;* (2) *health state, socioeconomic status, culture, and roles in family and community;* and (3) *maturity as a person.* These personal factors are the ones most likely to influence nurses' relations to patients. The age and sex differences between the patient and the nurse are of considerable importance. A male patient, for example, may be either willing or reluctant to accept assistance from a female nurse. Health and the changes that normally occur with aging may limit what nurses can do regardless of what they are willing to do. For these reasons some norms related to personal factors are specified as pertinent considerations in certain types of nursing positions.

A nurse's socioeconomic and cultural background may influence the requirements for socializing efforts in a given situation. Nurses must be cognizant of the similarities and differences between the patient's pattern of living and their own that may have an influence on both the patient and themselves. Some nurses have a tendency to look at certain patterns of living as inferior merely because these practices are different from their own or from their ideal.

The nurse's maturity as a person determines how he or she will perceive himself or herself and the patient within a helping relationship. Mature nurses have a realistic view of themselves. Family and community demands may exert a desirable or an undesirable influence upon a nurse. Lack of energy and interest, or preoccupation with matters outside the nursing situation, are some of the effects family and community demands may create. There are also positive effects; for example, the demands of family and community may stimulate the nurse's interest in people and in solving problems of living. Enlightened motivation and wisdom in helping and working with people in interpersonal situations are important positive effects that accrue to the mature nurse.

Included under nurse responsibilities are factors that, on the one hand, help to determine what the nurse is able to do and, on the other, what the nurse is permitted to do. Three groups of factors are suggested: (1) education and experience in nursing practice, (2) limitations set by the nurse's position and role as related to the patient, and (3) the status of the nurse as a responsible person.

Education and experience in nursing practice help to define what a nurse is able to do and what he or she can be expected to do. The system of nursing education that has evolved in the second half of the twentieth century provides education for a number of roles in nursing practice— professional, technical, and vocational. The experiences of a nurse and the pursuit of continuing education will determine in large part the degree of expertness attained. Expert nursing is dependent, of course, on the nurse's own development of the art of nursing, and this requires personal effort and guidance from expert nurse practitioners.

A nurse's abilities and limitations for designing, providing, and managing nursing care at any time arise from initial education, experience, continuing education, and developed nursing skills. No nurse can be expert in all types of nursing situations. Particular situations require specific knowledge and skills, and some situations require a depth of knowledge in a number of areas. Legal restrictions set by the nurse's license to practice also limit what the nurse can do. In nursing practice, what a nurse is able to do and permitted to do legally should be known by the nurse, by the health care institutions in which he or she works, and, in some nursing situations, by the nurse's patients. The nurse's case load of patients and the time allocation for their care should not be determined arbitrarily. Both should be determined in relation to the nursing requirements of the patients, the nurse's capabilities for nursing practice, and the nurse's expertness in particular types of nursing situations.

Nurses make judgments and decisions about themselves, their families, and their patients. The quality of the judgments and decisions they make gives expression to their personal commitments and their sense of responsibility in life situations. The state of personal moral development achieved by a nurse affects the characteristics of the decisions the nurse makes in nursing situations as well as in other situations. Nursing students should have learning experiences that will facilitate their moral development. Nurses in practice should examine the decisions they make in nursing situations in order to achieve understanding of themselves, the deliberate choices they made, their understanding of the options open at the times the choices were made, and the relationship between what they know and what they do. A nurse may know what should be done when particular conditions prevail in a nursing situation, but of vital concern to both nurse and patient is the actual decision the nurse makes.

Responsible nurses evaluate their own nursing performance in light of the patient's requirements for care. They seek and accept nursing supervision and strive to develop as nurses. They identify factors in nursing situations that interfere with patient progress and are able and unafraid to act to bring about change or represent these conditions to other responsible persons. Changes in nursing practice come about to the degree that nurses are both knowledgeable and responsible.

SELECTED READINGS

Backscheider, J. E.: "Self-Care Requirements, Self-Care Capabilities and Nursing Systems in the Diabetic Nurse Management Clinic," *American Journal of Public Health,* vol. 64, December 1974, pp. 1138–1146.

Bucher, Sue, and Joan G. Stelling: *Becoming Professional,* Sage Publications, Beverly Hills, Calif., 1977.

Burkett, Gary L.: "A Comparative Study of Physicians' and Nurses' Conceptions of the Role of Nurse Practitioners," *American Journal of Public Health,* vol. 68, November 1978, pp. 1090–1096.

Creighton, Helen (ed.): *Current Legal and Professional Issues: The Nursing Clinics of North America,* vol. 9, September 1974.

Foreman, Nancy Jo, and Joyce V. Zerwekh: "Drug Crisis Intervention," *American Journal of Nursing,* vol. 71, September 1971, pp. 1736–1739.

Gerdes, Lenore: "The Confused or Delirious Patient," *American Journal of Nursing,* vol. 68, June 1968, pp. 1228–1233.

Goulding, Erna I., and C. Everett Koop: "The Newborn, His Response to Surgery," *American Journal of Nursing,* vol. 66, August 1966, pp. 1762–1763.

Lewis, Barbara, and Cary L. Cooper: "Personality Measurement among Nurses: A Review," *International Journal of Nursing Studies,* vol. 13, 1976, pp. 209–229.

Piemme, J., and M. Trainor: "A First-Year Nursing Course in a Baccalaureate Program," *Nursing Outlook,* vol. 25, March 1977, pp. 184–187.

Pope, W., M. Reitz, and M. Patrick: "A Study of Oral Hygiene in the Geriatric Patient," *International Journal of Nursing Studies,* vol. 12, 1975, pp. 65–92.

Pridham, K. F.: "Instruction of a School-Age Child with Chronic Illness for Increased Responsibility in Self-Care, Using Diabetes Mellitus as an Example," *International Journal of Nursing Studies,* vol. 8, 1971, pp. 237–246.

Read, Donald A., Sidney B. Simon, and Joel B. Goodman: *Health Education: The Search for Values,* Prentice-Hall, Englewood Cliffs, N.J., 1977.

Roberts, Sharon L.: *Behavioral Concepts and the Critically Ill Patient,* Prentice-Hall, Englewood Cliffs, N.J., 1977.

Steele, Shirley M., and Vera M. Harmon: *Values Clarification in Nursing,* Appleton-Century-Crofts, New York, 1979.

Ventura, Marlene R.: "Related Social Behaviors of Students in Different Types of Nursing Education Programs," *International Journal of Nursing Studies,* vol. 13, 1976, pp. 3–10.

History

Hampton, Isabel A., et al.: *Nursing of the Sick 1893,* McGraw-Hill, New York, 1949.

Nightingale, Florence: *Notes on Nursing: What It Is, and What It Is Not,* J. B. Lippincott, Philadelphia, 1946.

Richards, Linda Ann Judson: *Reminiscences of Linda Richards, America's First Trained Nurse,* M. Barrows, Boston, 1911.

Staupers, Mabel Kenton: *No Time for Prejudice,* Macmillan, New York, 1961.

Thoms, Adah B. (ed.): *Pathfinders, A History of the Progress of Colored Graduate Nurses, with Biographies of Many Prominent Nurses,* Kay Printing House, New York, 1929.

Woolsey, Abby Howland: *A Century of Nursing, with Hints toward the Organization of a Training School, and Florence Nightingale's Historic Letter on the Bellevue School, September 18, 1872,* Putnam, New York, 1950.

Nursing and Health

NURSING, A FORM OF HEALTH CARE

Nursing is contributed effort toward designing, providing, and managing systems of therapeutic self-care for individuals or multiperson units within their daily living environments. Nursing's health dimension is derived from its self-care focus. Self-care, if it is to be positively therapeutic, helps to sustain life processes, to maintain integrated functioning, to promote normal growth and development, and to prevent or regulate disease and disability and their effects. The impending birth of a child, a construction worker's hospitalization after a fall from a building, a young man's paralysis sustained in an automobile accident, or a mother's prolonged illness are a few examples of some of the health-related situations in life that require the assistance of the nurse in helping an individual or family compensate for or overcome the limitations in self-care activities imposed by an existing health situation. The goal in nursing, like the goal in all other health services, is to achieve health results for individuals or groups, sick or well, when they need help. Commonly heard expressions describe quite clearly, if not in scientific terms, what is meant by health goals: "to stay well," "to get well," "to be cured," "to get stronger," "to get back to work," "to get over my nervousness," "to regain the use of my hand," "to have a healthy baby," "to have [Eddie] able to run and play again," and "to be able to live like other people again." These and similar expressions, heard many times a day by health care workers, describe the health goals sought by and for patients. They are associated with a movement of the patient away from abnormalities and the restriction of normal human activity due to disease, injury, or unsound relationships toward a goal of normalcy or wholeness. Health results sought for patients also may mean stabilizing the condition of a patient who is chronically ill or easing the suffering of the patient who is dying.

Health and *healthy* are terms used to describe living things—plants, animals, human beings—when they are structurally and functionally whole or sound. Individual human beings are said to be healthy or unhealthy. The same words are used to describe parts of the body, physiological mechanisms, control of emotional reactions, and mental functioning as well as attitudes and motives. Individuals evaluate their own states of integrity or wholeness, appraise each day, or sometimes more frequently, whether they feel well or sick. They also make judgments about the health of others with whom they have direct or even indirect contact. These evaluative judgments imply that individuals have ideas of what health means, at least to them, as well as ideas of the evidence needed to judge that a person is healthy or unhealthy.

In light of the complexity of human functioning and its relationships to environmental elements and conditions, *health* is a term that has considerable general utility in describing the state of wholeness or integrity of human beings. However, temporary indispositions such as not feeling well today, having a brief illness, or being injured do not necessarily place the individual in the unhealthy category. Some structural and functional changes do not seriously interfere with human integrated functioning or else interfere with it in a circumscribed fashion. For example, a healthy child or adult with a fracture of an extremity may feel well though not structurally or functionally whole because of the break in the bone and the limitations of movement. Individuals in this state would be referred to as "injured and disabled" rather than as "sick" or "in poor health." However, any deviation from normal structure or functioning is properly referred to as an absence of health in the sense of wholeness or integrity.

Human beings are distinguished from other living things by their capacity (1) to reflect upon themselves and their environment, (2) to symbolize what they experience, and (3) to use symbolic creations (ideas, words) in thinking, in communicating, and in guiding efforts to do and to make things that are beneficial for themselves or others. Health, then, must include that which makes a person human (form of mental life), operating in conjunction with physiological and psychophysiological mechanisms and a material structure (biologic life) and in relation to and interacting with other human beings (interpersonal and social life). The meaning of the term *health* changes as views about people's human and biological characteristics change.

Members of the health professions realize that they should be concerned with health in relation to integrated human functioning, including the contribution of their roles to its attainment. Nursing and the health professions are thus placed in a position where members must have knowledge from a number of different fields if they are to use and develop the health sciences and health technologies that are valid in bringing about the kinds of changes in human beings that move them toward, rather than away from, a state of wholeness, a state of human integrity. With the extension of the term *health* to include psychological, interpersonal, and social aspects of living as well as the commonly emphasized physical aspect, the health professions are beginning to recognize that, ideally, health is the responsibility of a society and its individual members and not of any one segment of that society.

The physical, psychological, interpersonal, and social aspects of health are inseparable in the individual. For example, consider a mother of several small children who has learned that she has tuberculosis. Her husband is employed full-time in a local factory and the family lives in a crowded flat in a large city. Her income from a part-time job has been important in providing some of the essential family needs. Her medical treatment, in addition to drug therapy, requires a prescribed amount of rest, a nutritious diet, and fresh air. The family's socioeconomic situation will affect the mother's ability to obtain the care she needs to arrest the tuberculosis. Her concern for her family and herself, in turn, will affect her mental state and thus her ability to rest and to participate in her own therapy. The maturity of the husband and wife, their creative abilities, the available resources they seek, and the support received from family members, friends, neighbors, and persons in the helping professions will affect the well-being of the family. The abilities of the husband and wife to cooperate and to coordinate their efforts toward designing and producing a system of effective self-care for the wife that is integrated with dependent-care systems for the children and the husband's self-care system will be a determining force in the provision of restorative health care for the mother and of primary preventive health care for the children and father.

Adversity in the form of ill health, scarcity of resources, or widespread disaster brings human suffering. But adversity may also bring people increased understanding of themselves and others. The human qualities of courage, patience or self-possession, and willingness to give of oneself to others are often revealed by people who suffer adversity.

The hypothetical example illustrates in a general way that various aspects of human functioning are interrelated. Accepting that an individual is an integrated whole is often difficult, perhaps because the sciences split humanity up; that is, they focus on different aspects of human structure or functioning to develop bodies of knowledge about human beings. Lay persons and health workers tend to think of the individual human being as having one part called a *body* and another part called a *mind*, with the two parts interacting. A more acceptable image is that a human being is a unity that can be viewed as functioning biologically, symbolically, and socially.

Deliberate action by adults to maintain a state of health for themselves and their dependents involves the components of self-care discussed in Chapter 3. Self-care as action requires a base of education in the home, at school, and from practical experiences in self-care. Self-care is only one aspect of healthful living, but without continuous self-care that has therapeutic quality, integrated human functioning will be disrupted. Good health habits are essential in maintaining health, but the ability to change old habits to meet new requirements may be as essential. Education in self-care, not just training in self-care practices, is necessary for the development of knowledge, skills, and positive attitudes related to self-care and health. Children, adolescents, and young adults have interests in health and health care. All too frequently, adults with whom young people have contact are unable, unwilling, or uninterested in providing adequate help. In modern society parents and other educators should be concerned with what can be done to enable children to learn to direct themselves toward a state of integrated functioning and well-being that would promote human dignity and beauty even in illness and disability.

HEALTH AS A STATE

Dictionaries as well as the World Health Organization, an agency of the United Nations, use the term *state* in defining health. Human health or well-being is defined as "the state of being whole or sound." Although the word *health* is especially used to refer to the state of being free from "physical disease or pain," it is also used to refer to "soundness of mind and soul." The World Health Organization emphasizes that health is a state of physical, mental, and social well-being and not merely the absence of disease or infirmity. To conceptualize health it is necessary to explore the term *state* in relationship to being sound or whole.

The term *state* applied to people is defined as the way a person reveals his or her existence. *State* is used in a very general fashion when applying it to any well-defined conditions of a person that are considered as a whole without specification or analysis of components, for example, the states of being calm or anxious, asleep or awake, acutely ill, debilitated, depressed. *State* is also defined as a compound state. The term is used in this sense, for example, when a person's health state is expressed as a set of determined values of specified human characteristics that simultaneously reveal some aspects of the person's existence. The specified characteristics are worked with as a compound entity (a vector) having a definite number of components, which, when taken together as a set, describe the state of the person at a particular time.

Examples of the use of the term *state* in the health field in the sense of compound state include the taking of the vital signs of temperature, pulse, respiration, and blood pressure and considering these together as an index of the state of selected vital processes. The component parts of and the findings of a complete or partial physical examination can be considered a compound entity useful in specifying an individual's health state to some desired completeness.[1] Since the usefulness of the vital signs or physical examination findings may differ from time to time, it is necessary to monitor events or seek evidence of characteristics during a particular time period to have knowledge of (1) the actual frequencies of the occurrence of events and (2) their determinate probabilities.[2]

The term *sound* means possession of full vigor and strength and the absence of signs of disease and morbidity. The term *whole* means that nothing has been omitted, ignored, or lessened. These terms, when used together in regard to health, signify human functional and structural integrity, absence of genetic defects, and progressive integrated development of a human being as an individual unity moving toward higher and higher levels of integration.[3] Each human being as a complex unity is often described as having physical, psychic, and intellectual characteristics that become more highly integrated with progressive development. It is obvious that health, defined as a state of being sound or whole, is a state of human perfection that includes continuing human development. It is also obvious that bodies of accumulated knowledge about humankind are necessary for making determinations of the health states of individuals. Furthermore, time-oriented norms are required if judgments are to be made about structural, functional, and genetic integrity and about human development.

A person's general appearance is often the basis used for making judgments about the person's health state, for example, making the judgment that this or that person appears to be in good or poor health or that his or her health has improved or worsened. A scientific appraisal of an

[1]W. Ross Ashby, *An Introduction to Cybernetics*, Chapman & Hall, Ltd., London, 1956, p. 30.
[2]Bernard J. F. Lonergan, *Insight*, Philosophical Library, New York, 1958, pp. 65–66.
[3]Ibid., pp. 469–479.

individual's health state requires that the term *state* be used in the compound sense. This approach necessitates that persons with the requisite knowledge search out the sets of human characteristics that will be useful in specifying health state to some desired completeness. Within the health field, biologists and physicians have contributed substantial bodies of knowledge about the physical aspects of human health. Norms have been established and approaches to determining anatomical, physiological, genetic, and psychophysiological components of the health state have been developed and refined (including specifying the kinds of information needed, data-gathering techniques, and rules for inference).

Psychic and intellectual components of an individual's health state viewed in the compound sense include (1) inner experiences, (2) behaviors and conduct (deliberate action) that can be observed in interpersonal and group situations, and (3) solitary endeavors. Concepts of mental health are not as firmly structured as those of physical health. Physical examinations, psychological tests, and the eliciting of subjective information from individuals about their behavior in interpersonal and group situations are used as means for obtaining information as a basis for making judgments about health states along these mental health dimensions. The development and use of these means is apportioned among a number of disciplines.

Health workers, including nurses, obtain and use information that describes and explains selected aspects of human structure and functioning. For example, nurses will use information obtained and expressed in terms of the disciplines of physiology and pathology in making judgments about self-care requisites and self-care agency of patients. Nurses are responsible for defining the components that describe health states of individuals and the quality and quantity of information about these components that are sufficient for nursing purposes. In order to deal with the many kinds of information obtainable about human developments and structural and functional states, some nurses and other health workers use the concept of "field," as Kurt Lewin defined it with respect to the life space of an individual or group.[4] Field theory is essentially a method useful in analyzing relationships and organizing information. Those who use this approach must identify and describe the component parts of the field (the vector) that they are examining.

When health is described as a state of being whole and sound, it is necessary to link human growth and development to human structure and functioning. A person's state of growth and development changes over time. At a specific time, a person will exhibit a degree of structural and functional integrity according to his or her stage of development. Genetic

[4]Kurt Lewin, in Dorian Cartwright (ed.), *Field Theory in Social Science,* Harper Torchbooks, New York, 1951, p. xi and p. 45

factors can affect the development as well as the structural and functional integrity of individuals.

For nursing purposes, it is more practical (1) to recognize that at any one time an individual has reached a particular stage of development, which means that certain developments have occurred or are occurring and that specific developments are or are not in accord with established norms and (2) then to attend to the person's functional and structural integrity. For this reason, and for purposes of this text, health state and developmental state are considered as separate entities. Nurses often *assume* that the developments of a person of a particular age are in accord with norms, for example, accepting the mature appearance of an individual as a basis for the judgment that he or she is mature. If a nurse *observes*, for example, that an individual cannot read or write, the nurse begins to examine various developments (e.g., cognitive developments) in order to know how to help the person understand and deal with meeting his or her therapeutic self-care demand.

For practical reasons, members of the various health professions must be able to take an approach to the health of individuals that will enable them to fulfill their purposes as health professionals in the social group. Ideally, members of the health professions view persons for whom they provide care as complex unities but view the possible components of the health states of individuals from the perspectives of their own disciplines. This means that they know the components to which they should attend and the meaning these components have for their own specialized work.

Throughout life, individuals tend to learn that some combination of components usually will serve them well as an index of their health state. Persons with certain diseases and those under certain forms of medical diagnosis or therapy must learn to collect data as a basis for judging their own human functioning. Learning to determine and determining what combination of components will serve as an index of health state may be a part of the patient role in health care situations. Nurses should seek information about how patients perceive their own health states and the meanings they attach to these states or to various components.

NURSING AND THE REGULATION OF HEALTH STATE

The points where nursing converges on the health state of an individual can be described in terms of self-care, self-care requisites, therapeutic self-care demand, the constituent elements of self-care agency, and the performance of self-care operations. Self-care has been described as deliberate action that enables the individual to survive in a variety of states of well-being or health or to move from one state to another. The person who has self-care agency and activates it in the performance of particular self-care operations can be said to be a *regulator*.[5] Such a person is a good regulator if his or her self-care actions bring about internal and external conditions necessary to maintain life processes and environmental conditions supportive of life processes, integrity of human structure and functioning, and human developmental processes.

Self-care actions selected from a therapeutic self-care demand are deliberately performed; they can be reproduced from one time to another; and they are selected and performed with the goal of keeping internal and external conditions constant according to some standard. The universal, developmental, and health-deviation self-care requisites are expressions of the types of regulatory actions that should be performed by self-care or dependent-care agents. Identification and description of types of self-care requisites supply nurses, other health workers, and the public with what is important and what is wanted with respect to regulation. The calculation of an individual's therapeutic self-care demand provides information about regulatory actions, which would ideally be performed because of the known values of selected health state components and the probability of constancy or change in these values.

Information about the values of health state components and the probabilities attached to their values allows nurses to make judgments about the current and projected effects of these components on the individual's performance of self-care operations. Furthermore, such information provides nurses with knowledge about conditions that require the use of particular helping methods in order to meet self-care requisites and to regulate the exercise or development of self-care agency. Nurses should also seek information about the cognitive and moral development of individuals, since it is significant for the development of the constituent parts of self-care agency and for their exercise in performing self-care operations. One broad index of health (including development) is an individual's view of self as a self-care or dependent-care agent and the freedom with which the individual accepts and acts with responsibility in matters of self-care or dependent care.

Achieving Health Results

Achieving health results is the goal for all health care services. The health results sought by and for individuals in our society are (1) to maintain a state of health, (2) to regain a normal or near normal state of health in the event of disease or injury, and (3) to stabilize, control, and minimize the effects of chronic poor health or disability. Workers in each health care service have specific roles in achieving health results. For example, physicians determine the presence or absence of disease or injury. They also prescribe or give care that enables the patient to maintain or regain a

[5]W. Ross Ashby, *An Introduction to Cybernetics*, Chapman & Hall, Ltd., London, 1956, pp. 195–218.

normal or near normal state of health. Laboratory technicians examine blood, urine, or tissue specimens. Their findings enable physicians to better diagnose the presence or absence of disease. X-ray technicians prepare x-ray film for similar purposes. Dietitians supervise the preparation of special or restricted diets as required in the treatment or control of disease. The nurse's part is specified and limited by nursing's focus on helping individuals to achieve health results through therapeutic self-care when its need is brought about by poor health or specialized requirements for health care. The nature and extent of a person's inabilities for engagement in self-care, the nature and numbers of self-care requisites, and the factors that limit how these requisites can be met determine the amount and kind of nursing that will be needed.

The provision of health services has become increasingly complex with the broadening concept of health, with advances in the sciences and in technology, and with the increasing numbers of health care workers and supportive and administrative personnel. Achieving health results for individuals, families, and communities within health services as presently organized is costly and often inefficient for the providers as well as the seekers and receivers of service. Financing health services, availability of services needed, quality of health care provided, communications among health workers, and coordination of services are some of the problem areas. The public as well as the organized health services must become more involved in finding solutions to problems in the delivery of health services in order to avoid serious breakdowns in service, to provide service when and where it is not presently available, and to improve the quality of service where this is needed. Nurses must continue, and in some instances begin, to assume their part in this effort.

NURSING AS HEALTH CARE

Nursing practice as related to individuals has become fixed or institutionalized around the process of one person (the nurse) giving direct help to another person (the patient) when that person is wholly or partly unable to help himself or herself in the accomplishment of daily health-related care because of the existing health situation. This help includes medically prescribed therapy in the treatment of disease and injury that is part of the patient's daily self-care. Nursing, then, is a helping or assisting service to persons who are wholly or partly dependent—infants, children, and adults—when they, their parents, guardians, or other adults responsible for their care are no longer able to give or supervise their care because of the nature of their therapeutic self-care needs.

Every nurse must be qualified to provide nursing to individuals, adults, or children who have demands for nursing assistance. As a helping art, nursing is the complex ability to accomplish or to contribute to the accomplishment of a person's usual and therapeutic self-care by compensating for or aiding in overcoming the conditions or disabilities that cause the person (1) to be unable to act, (2) to refrain from acting, or (3) to act ineffectively in self-care. From the viewpoint of the patient, nursing care is always something received; it is personal assistance or help from a person who is qualified and able to help. From the viewpoint of the nurse, however, nursing care is help effectively given. It is caring for, assisting with, or doing something for the patient to achieve the health results sought by and for the patient.

Nursing is referred to as *assistance* for two reasons. First, it is always something provided for another, and second, what is accomplished directly or indirectly through nursing, that is, the therapeutic self-care of the patient, is the responsibility of the one assisted under normal conditions. Ideally, the nurse regards himself or herself and behaves as the assister, or assistant, in every nursing situation. Nurses direct their efforts, guided by a nursing focus, toward achieving the health results sought for the patient. As an assistant, a helper to the patient, the nurse should never lose sight of the patient's ultimate responsibility for his or her own self-care or, in the case of a child patient, the responsibility of the parents or guardian for caring for and guiding the child in the maintenance of health through self-care.

The Nursing Focus versus the Medical Focus

Healthy adults perform many of the universal components of self-care without direct help. They feed, wash, dress, and perform many health-related actions for themselves, including seeking medical care when they recognize the need for it. These and other activities usually become a fixed part of daily living and are scarcely noticed. The sick or injured adult, however, may find that he or she is unable to accomplish usual self-care tasks. The universal components of self-care may have to be modified because of an individual's health situation. The person may have little or no knowledge about the new care components that are required because of illness or injury. The person requires nursing assistance, and the nurse contributes to his or her well-being by providing that assistance. The following example demonstrates the focus of nursing and the part the nurse shares with others in achieving health results for patients.

A man has sustained serious burns of the face, neck, chest, and arms. He is suffering considerable pain, and certain movements intensify his pain. He is very ill. Some of his body tissues have been destroyed; he is extremely anxious about his condition; he fears disfigurement, disability, and even death. He does not question his hospitalization, his need for medical care, or his wife's continuous presence. He accepts without question the ministrations of the attending doctors and nurses, including the pain they may unavoidably cause him as they care for him. The doctors and nurses know their roles in assisting him. They have learned what they must do for him and how to do it most effectively through specialized education and training. This knowledge includes medical knowledge of burns and treatment techniques; a background knowledge of anatomy and physiology, chemistry, microbiology, pharmacology, nutrition, psychology, and sociology; and experience in observing and working under the supervision of experienced doctors and nurses who were caring for burn patients.

The focus of the nurse's activities in this example is the man with burns who requires assistance to prevent further deterioration of his health and to recover and return to his normal or a near normal way of life. But the doctor has the same focus for his or her activities. What then is specific to the nursing objectives for the patient? First, one must look closely at the interests shared by doctor and nurse. Both see the patient as a human being—as a person who is unique, who has rights and responsibilities for himself and others, who has motives and values, and who has a way of life that has been disrupted by his accident and his present states of illness and dependency. Both see the patient as they see other members of the human race—as a rational living being, vulnerable to disease and injury, but with great capacity to combat disease and injury, to recover, or to adjust and find ways for compensating for lost abilities and to be courageous in so doing.

The doctor's special interests in this situation are the patient's life processes as they have been disrupted as a result of the burns. They may be further disrupted by improper or careless treatment, by invading microorganisms resulting in infection, and by failure to support the patient psychologically and help him sustain his will to live during the initial and critical phase of his illness and in the recovery phase when disfigurement must be faced. The doctor is specially prepared to evaluate the physical and psychophysical aspects of the patient's condition and progress and to prescribe appropriate therapeutic measures to prevent or alleviate complications that may develop.

The nurse's special interest is the continuing therapeutic care the patient requires. The nurse is concerned with the universal components of self-care, now modified by the burns and their effects upon the man's integrated functioning, and with all the health-deviation components of care that may arise as a result of the burns. The nurse assists the patient on a continuous basis with his personal care, which he can no longer manage for himself, and sustains him during the periods of great suffering and mental stress resulting from his pain and fear.

The nursing focus takes into account both the medical point of view and the patient's point of view. The doctor's prescribed measures for the treatment and control of the patient's condition will have been instituted promptly as a part of the patient's continuing care, as well as other measures designed to aid the doctor in diagnosing and instituting early treatment to prevent complications. The doctor, however, requires information about the physiological and behavioral state of the patient during the time he or she is not present to observe them. Continuing observation and recordings of the patient's condition throughout each day are important components of therapeutic care made necessary by the patient's specific health situation. The nurse must be alert to the patient's condition to adjust care to immediate needs, including the possibility of a need for immediate or emergency medical care because of a worsening of the patient's condition.

Recognizing an emergency situation and securing immediate medical assistance is an important component of self-care that the patient in the example can no longer manage for himself. It necessarily becomes a part of the nursing focus. The patient may not be aware of his need for observation. He may not even be able to recognize his need for emergency medical assistance. The nursing focus, from the patient's point of view, requires recognition and acceptance by the nurse that it is the patient who is living with his burned tissues, that it is the patient who must cope with the effects of physiological changes and of fear and pain on his integrity as an individual. The patient perceives his situation. He thinks about the future. He imagines what it may be, and he is afraid. A nursing focus is unrealistic if it does not take into account how the patient views and is personally affected by his illness. The nurse's recognition and acceptance of the patient's point of view is essential if the patient is to be assisted through nursing to live with his illness and disability, to cooperate with those who assist him, and above all to be motivated to direct his energies toward recovering a normal or near normal state of health.

Parts of the Nursing Focus

There are six components of a nursing focus. These components include the physician's perspective and the patient's perspective of the health situation and four central patient components: (1) state of health, (2) health results sought, (3) the therapeutic self-care demand, and (4) present abilities and disabilities to engage in self-care. The parts of a nursing focus and their interrelationship are shown in Fig. 6-1.

Each of the six components shown is in itself complex. Both the physician's medical perspective of the patient's health state and health care needs and the patient's perspective of his or her health situation should be seen as encompassing all or parts of each of the four central patient components. The four patient components are complex and interrelated. Both physician and nurse contribute to the identification and

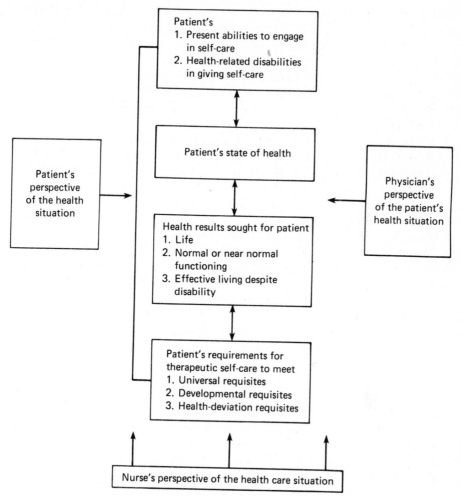

Figure 6-1 The parts of a nursing focus.

delineation of these components, and this requires securing and validating information about the patient's health state and heath-derived requirements for health care. The patient's health state not only gives rise to requirements for health care, it also affects the patient's ability to engage in self-care activities.

The foundation for the basic design of a system of nursing for a patient is determined by identifying and describing the nursing focus for the patient. The parts of the nursing focus and their interrelationships are the elements from which the nursing design is formed. The design changes as the components change; for example, as a patient's health state improves, the health-deviation self-care requisites may decrease and self-care ability increase, thus increasing the patient's self-care activities and decreasing the number of care activities that nurses perform for the patient. Identification and description of the six components of the nursing focus and their interrelationships for individual patients make explicit the *health dimension of nursing* for each patient. This information serves to guide the nurse in maintaining a nursing perspective on the patient that is defined in health terms.

In developing a nursing perspective, the components of the nursing focus become the guides for nursing action to the degree that the nurse understands each component, acquires information relating to it in specific nursing situations, and is able to interpret this information and attach nursing meaning to it. Consider a healthy adult woman who has sustained a fracture of a lower extremity and is immobilized in a cast. The patient is unable to do many things for herself because of her lack of mobility. The nursing focus in this situation should consider the patient's lack of mobility in its relationship to her general state of health and the health results sought. It will be clear to the nurse, in the light of nursing knowledge, that nonuse of the fractured extremity is both a component of the patient's therapeutic self-care and the underlying cause of the patient's inability to perform other usual self-care measures. It will also be clear that, objectively, the health results sought are (1) the healing of the fracture, (2) a return of the normal functioning of the extremity, and (3) the patient's recovery of mobility. The health results sought, however, are in turn directly related to and depend upon the patient's age, general state of health, nutritional state, and physiological capacity for forming the new bone growth necessary to the healing of the fracture. (The physiological capacity for forming new bone tissue is frequently reduced in aged or undernourished patients.) The physician may view the patient's health situation primarily from an orthopedic point of view, with a primary concern for the effectiveness of the method of immobilization used and other aspects of the therapeutic regimen to promote healing. The patient may be primarily concerned with the effects of the fracture—pain, discomfort, disability, disruption of activities, and with the probable duration of the treatment.

When nurses enter nursing relationships with patients, they must distill from the mass of patient characteristics those that are relevant to the nursing focus. Nurses do not ignore the nonrelevant factors but view them in light of the influence they may exert on the factors that determine the specifications for nursing action. Further, nurses must keep in mind that the nursing focus for a patient may be either relatively stable or undergoing continuous change. In the earlier example of the patient with severe burns, the nursing focus probably would require adjustment from hour to hour, or even more frequently, during the critical periods of the patient's illness. The frequency of change in the physician's perspective, as well as in the patient's perspective, during these critical periods would necessarily affect the nursing perspective as well. Changes in the nursing perspective probably would occur less frequently after stabilization of the patient's condition, but the nurse would need to know and understand how change in one component of the nursing focus would affect the other components. For example, if there is a sudden and dramatic improvement in the burn patient's condition, or if he suffers a sudden relapse and becomes comatose, his requirements for therapeutic care and his ability to engage in self-care would change dramatically. The sudden change in one component of the nursing focus (the patient's state of health) may set off a chain reaction in all the other components that would make it essential for the nurse to completely revise the nursing focus for the patient.

The nursing focus is also the index or key in estimating the complexity of a nursing situation and thus in determining the kinds of nurses (e.g., level of education and training) that will be needed to meet the patient's requirements for nursing care. The complexity of a nursing situation is determined by (1) the rapidity of change in the components of the nursing focus, (2) the elements of the components, and (3) the number and kinds of relationships between the components. The complexity of a nursing situation is increased whenever the nursing focus is not clear-cut or obvious, for example, a situation in which the patient is critically ill but the reasons for the illness are unknown. A clear-cut or obvious nursing focus is one that can be validly established by means of readily available information about the components and their relationships.

The ability to develop and maintain a valid nursing focus in nursing practice is directly related to the nurse's educational preparation and experience. The mark of the expert in nursing is the ability to see a health care situation from a nursing perspective and to recognize personal capabilities and limitations in establishing and maintaining a valid nursing focus. Because of limitations in their educational preparation, some nurses are not prepared to design, establish, and maintain a valid system of nursing for a patient without the supervision of a nurse with advanced preparation and experience. These same nurses, however, may be qualified by their educational background and well prepared to work in cooperation with another nurse, or they may be prepared to care for a patient in keeping with a design preestablished and maintained by another qualified nurse.

REQUIREMENTS FOR HEALTH CARE

Health care is based on systems of knowledge about health and disease and on practices with some demonstrated value in promoting health or in preventing, curing, or regulating disease. Concepts descriptive of systems of *preventive health care* are useful in unifying the meaning of health, disease, and health care for individuals. For this reason prevention is the concept used as the means for presenting and interpreting variations of health care requirements and their meaning in nursing situations. Prevention as described by Leavell, Clark, and others is based on (1) knowledge of the natural history of human disorders, (2) knowledge of the combination of causes of specific disorders of human structure and functioning, and (3) an identified rational basis for methods of intercepting or counteracting causative factors before the onset of a disease or at some period after its onset.[6] Preventive health care thus requires knowledge of specific interferences with normal human structure and functioning at various stages of the life cycle in particular environments.

Systems of preventive health care recognize three levels of prevention: primary, secondary, and tertiary. Primary prevention is appropriate before the onset of disease and is directed to the *maintenance and promotion of health* and the *prevention of specific deseases*. Secondary prevention is appropriate after the onset of disease and is directed to the *prevention of complications* (disease that occurs concurrently with other disease) and of *sequelae* (disorders of structure or function that follow or are caused by an attack of a disease) and *prevention of prolonged disability*. Tertiary prevention is appropriate when there is disability with a demand to function in society with limited human capacities. It is directed toward bringing about *effective and satisfying human functioning in accord with existing powers for human functioning*. The reader should refer to works in preventive medicine for detailed explanations of these levels of prevention.

Requirements of individuals for the three levels of preventive health care vary with age, states of development and health, and external environmental conditions. Care at the primary level of prevention is a requirement of each individual throughout life. With the onset of disease or when a person is disabled, there will be requirements for care at the secondary and tertiary levels of prevention. Each person in a health care situation can be viewed therefore as having one of the following kinds of preventive health care requirements:

1 Care at the primary level of prevention
2 Care at the primary and secondary levels of prevention
3 Care at the primary and tertiary levels of prevention
4 Care at the primary, secondary, and tertiary levels of prevention

These four kinds of health care requirements have meaning for nursing because of their implications for life, health, and effective living on the

---

[6] Hugh Rodman Leavell, E. Gurney Clark, et al., *Preventive Medicine for the Doctor in His Community*, 3d ed., McGraw-Hill, New York, 1965, pp. 14–38.

part of the patient and the health care role responsibilities that each level of care specifies for patients, health workers, and others who provide care and services. They further impose demands for specific attitudes, knowledge, and skills on the part of patients, health workers, or others who provide care and services. Each level of prevention is considered so that some implications for nursing are made explicit.

Health Care Requirements at the Primary Level of Prevention

Requirements for health maintenance and promotion and disease prevention are specified in relation to what is known about (1) human structure and functioning and (2) specific diseases or interferences with the normal human condition. The effective meeting of the universal self-care requisites adjusted to age, environmental conditions, and the individual's health and developmental state is health care at the primary level of prevention.

The adult has a major instrumental role in health care at the primary level of prevention because it is a continuous requirement. When the person is young, aged, ill, unknowing, or unskilled, the role of agent for meeting that person's universal self-care requisites should be taken by a responsible and qualified adult. The nurse may be this adult or may help another adult fill the role competently. The physician's or dentist's role is that of diagnostician in periodic health examinations, prescriber of preventive therapy (for example, diet adjusted to age), or instrumental agent in giving preventive therapy (e.g., specific preventive therapy after exposure to but before the onset of a specific communicable disease). The community role in health care at the primary level of prevention is a large one and relates to control of environmental conditions and adequacy of essential resources. It provides health services in the form of education to prepare individuals and families to fulfill their personal care roles. It also provides private or public health services to protect individuals from specific disease or to help them with problems of health maintenance and promotion.

General rules to guide nurses in identifying some of the nursing dimensions of health care requirements at the primary level of prevention include the following:

1 Every individual under nursing care has health care requirements at the primary level of prevention.

2 Universal self-care and developmental self-care (Chapter 3), when therapeutic in quality, constitute health care at the primary level of prevention. They include practices to maintain and promote health and development and to prevent specific diseases. Practices to promote health are based on rationales of resources and conditions essential for survival and development and for normalcy of structure and functioning. Practices to prevent specific diseases are based on rationales of how to prevent or interrupt relations between causative agents of disease and factors in patients or the environment that together establish the conditions necessary for the disease to develop.

3 In assisting individual patients, nurses are able to select and use or guide patients to select and use methods for meeting self-care requisites that promote and maintain health and development and prevent specific disease. Methods are properly adjusted to the factors of age, health, individual modes of functioning, and environment.

4 Nurses apply factual information about the patient, the environment, the patient's life-style, and routine of daily living in their selection or use of universal and developmental self-care practices at the primary level of prevention. Health care at this level should be incorporated into each patient's system of daily living and be a permanent part of it.

5 Nurses assist patients in health care directed to the goals of health maintenance and promotion and disease prevention with an awareness of the essential role of the patient or a responsible adult in the continuous provision of this level of preventive health care.

Health Care Requirements at the Secondary and Tertiary Levels of Prevention

Requirements for (1) prevention of complicating diseases and adverse effects of specific diseases and prolonged disability through early diagnosis and treatment (secondary prevention) and (2) rehabilitation in the event of disfigurement and disability (tertiary level of prevention) are specified in relation to what is known about the nature and effects of specific diseases, valid methods of regulating disease, and the human potential for living with and overcoming the disabling effects of disease. Health-deviation self-care of a therapeutic quality includes practices at either or both of these levels of prevention.

Health care at the secondary level of prevention is accomplished through accurate diagnosis and effective treatment at the onset or in some later stage of a disease. Periodic health examinations, accurate observation of signs and symptoms of health disorders by patient, family, or nurse, and the selection of further health care as indicated by observed signs and symptoms facilitate early diagnosis and treatment when adequate medical services are available. Case finding in public health practice also facilitates early diagnosis and treatment.

During the course of a disease process, health care requirements and the instrumental role of the patient as self-care agent vary with the effects of the disease and with the methods of diagnosis and treatment used. Health care is effective at the secondary level of prevention if (1) the disease is cured, the pathological process arrested, or the effects of the disease kept under control, (2) complicating diseases are prevented, and (3) the dissemination of the causative agents of the disease is prevented.

Rehabilitation, as previously indicated, requires deliberate action on the part of the patient and health workers to adapt or adjust functioning to compensate for or overcome disabilities that restrict human functioning in specific ways. Rehabilitative health care varies with the nature and the effects of the disability, including the stage of the life cycle when the disabling condition occurred. It also varies with the methods used for determining the extent of the disability, the patient's remaining functional capacity, and the techniques used to enable the patient to function effectively with some degree of satisfaction. This level of health care requires a belief in the human potential to overcome disability, effective techniques for determining functional loss and remaining functional capacities, and effective restorative or compensatory techniques. It also requires willingness on the part of the patient, the family, health workers, and communities to work toward the goal of rehabilitation. Many types of specialists and provisions for special education, recreation, travel, and work must be available on a community basis. This level of preventive health care is effective whenever an individual is able to live or is making progress in living as an active member of a social group.

General rules to guide nurses in identifying the nursing dimensions of situations where patients have requirements for the secondary or tertiary levels of preventive health care include the following:

1   Persons who suffer from disease or disorders of health or their effects have health care requirements at the secondary or tertiary levels of prevention that are specific to an active disease process (or processes) and its continuous dynamic effects or to a state of disfigurement or dysfunction.

2   Health-deviation self-care (Chapter 3), when therapeutic in quality, is health care at the secondary or tertiary level of prevention in the form of self-care measures to regulate and prevent adverse effects of the disease, prevent complicating diseases, prevent prolonged disability, or adapt or adjust functioning to overcome or compensate for the adverse effects of permanent or prolonged disfigurement or dysfunction.

3   In assisting individual patients, nurses must be able to use and to guide patients in the use of medically prescribed or endorsed measures of diagnosis, treatment, and rehabilitation to be incorporated into self-care, including adjustments of universal and developmental self-care requisites to the health and disease state of the patient.

4   Nurses gather and apply factual information about the patient, including results of medical evaluations that specify level of functioning measured against norms for healthy individuals in the patient's age group, medical orders, environment, life-style, and routines of daily living.

5   Health care at these levels becomes a temporary or a permanent part of a patient's daily life.

6   Nurses assist patients in health care directed to the goals of sec-

ondary and tertiary prevention with the awareness that the role of the patient as responsible instrumental agent in health care varies not only with age but also with the nature of the disease process and its effects. It also varies with the measures and techniques of diagnosis, treatment, and rehabilitation used in health care, their effects on the patient, the resources and services available to the patient, and his or her state of readiness to give or manage self-care with or without guidance and supervision.

CLASSIFICATION OF NURSING SITUATIONS BY HEALTH FOCUS

Since the same totality of things, persons, or situations may be classified in more than one way, it is necessary to consider the methods of establishing classifications. For example, if one has a box of red and yellow beads and if some of these beads are round and the others square, the beads may be grouped according to color or to shape. The groupings are red beads and yellow beads when classified by color and round beads and square beads when classified by shape. If some red beads and some yellow beads are round and others square, then it is possible to group them according to both schemes of classification by placing red ones into separate groups of round and square beads and yellow ones into similar groups.

Classification is useful not only in organizing information or facts but also in serving practical purposes. In practical endeavors, considering each of the varying factors (e.g., color and shape of the beads) is necessary whenever the variations have an effect on the desired result. For a very simple example, consider that the red and yellow beads in the box are to be used in making two necklaces of the following design—beads of the same color, alternating round and square beads. Both color and shape must be considered in the planning. The number of round and square beads of each color for making two necklaces of specific lengths must be determined. Size of the beads and the number of beads available are other relevant considerations. Arrangement of the beads into two color groups and of each color group into two shape groups would facilitate making judgments about the number of beads available as well as stringing the beads. This simple example of the beads illustrates how classifications are developed in terms of characteristics and how useful classification is in identifying and naming things and in accomplishing a task or a series of tasks. To function effectively, nurses require knowledge of both the health and helping aspects of nursing situations. A classification system that would assist nurses in understanding the health aspects of nursing situations is presented below.

A Suggested Classification of Nursing Situations

A person in need of nursing care can be described from a health perspective with reference to (1) the presence or absence of disease, injury, disability, or disfigurement; (2) the quality of general health state described in the general sense as excellent, good, fair, poor, or in terms of the values of sets of selected characteristics that together define the person's health state; and (3) the life-cycle-oriented events and circumstances that indicate current changes and existing needs for health care. These dimensions of health, when accurately described for a patient, indicate appropriate health care goals, specify the kinds of health care required, and may also indicate the kinds of obstacles to self-care that are present or could be present. A classification system based on these dimensions of health is suggested, and seven groupings of nursing situations according to the health focus of the situation are proposed. The suggested variations in each group identify subgroups. The classification is generally useful, that is, not just useful to nurses. It is essentially a classification of health care situations from which inferences about the nursing aspects of health care can be made.

Group 1   The health focus is oriented to events and circumstances in relation to the *life cycle* that give rise to anatomical, physiological, or psychological changes associated with periods of growth and development, maturity, parenthood, the process of aging, and the period of old age. General health is within the range of excellent to good.

Group 2   The health focus is oriented to the process of *recovery* from a specific disease (e.g., measles) or injury (e.g., a fracture of the pelvis resulting from a fall) or to overcoming or compensating for the effects of the disease or injury. Permanent *disfigurement* or *disability* may or may not be present or expected. General health is within the range of excellent to good.

Group 3   The health focus is oriented to *illness or disorder of undetermined origin,* with concern for the degree of illness, specific effects of the disorder, and effects of specific diagnostic or therapeutic measures used. General health is within the range of good to fair.

Group 4   The health focus is oriented to *defects of a genetic or developmental nature* or to the *biological state of the premature infant* or the infant of *low birth weight*. The state of general health is or may be affected by the direct or indirect effects of the defect or the biological state.

Group 5   The health focus is oriented to *regulation through active treatment of a disease or disorder or injury of determined origin,* with concern for the degree of illness, the specific effects of the disease, disorder, or injury, and the specific effects of the therapeutic measures used. Temporary or permanent disfigurement or disability may or may not be present or expected. The state of general health is or may be affected by direct or indirect effects of the disease, disorder, or injury.

Group 6   The health focus is oriented to the *restoration, stabilization, or regulation of integrated functioning.* A vital process may have stopped or be seriously disrupted, or, in a newborn infant, breathing may not have started.

Group 7   The health care focus is oriented to the regulation of the effects of processes that have disrupted human integrated functioning to the degree that life cannot long continue. Rational processes may be disturbed or relatively unaffected.

VARIATIONS IN HEALTH CARE AND NURSING

Each of the seven groupings of nursing situations, because of differences in health focus, indicates requirements for different kinds of combinations of health care directed to one or more of the goals of preventive health care. For example, in nursing situations with a life cycle focus, the requirement for health care is at the primary level of prevention with the goals of maintaining and promoting health and preventing specific diseases and injuries. Awareness of these goals guides nurses as well as other health workers in the selection of measures of care and assistance for individuals or groups within specific environments.

In the descriptions that follow, health care goals and health care needs are specified and variations indicated for each health focus. It should be understood that while the life cycle orientation to health care represents a type of nursing situation, in nursing practice the guides suggested for care with this focus are used along with guides for each of the other six situations, since every person is in one of the phases of the life cycle. The life cycle focus validates and provides the base for both universal and developmental self-care requisites. Health-deviation self-care requisites are associated with groups 2 to 6. The helping focus of nursing must be linked to the health care focus (see Fig. 6-2). The linking of the helping and health focuses in nursing practice is mediated by patient variables, therapeutic self-care demand and self-care agency, and the relationship between them.

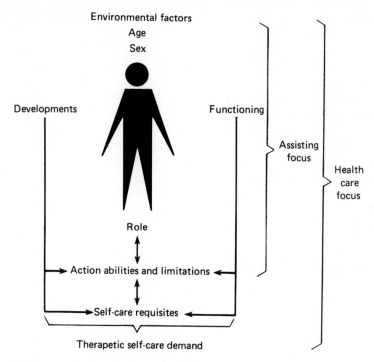

Environmental factors
Age
Sex

Developments

Functioning

Assisting
focus

Health
care
focus

Role

Action abilities and limitations

Self-care requisites

Therapetic self-care demand

Figure 6-2 Two focuses of nurses in health care situations.

Life Cycle

In a nursing situation where the health focus is oriented to the life cycle, the care is designed for promoting and maintaining health and for protecting against specific diseases and injuries. Environmental conditions and internal changes connected with intrauterine growth and development, infancy, childhood, adolescence, and maturity and related events and conditions such as pregnancy, menopause, and aging determine the specific kinds of health care that will be needed.

A nursing case of this type is one in which the patient's behavior indicates well-being rather than illness and in which there is evidence that the patient is in good to excellent health. The general health care needs would include:

1 Periodic health evaluation to determine the normalcy of the patient's growth, functioning, and development, and the quality of general health

2 Health maintenance and promotion adjusted to the specific phase of and events in the patient's life cycle and to general health

3 Protection against environmental factors, with specific concern for growth and development
4 Assistance to the patient and the family in assuming appropriate roles in continuing health care through self-care

When the health focus is oriented to the life cycle, therapeutic self-care consists primarily of meeting the universal and developmental components of self-care adjusted to age, to sex, to the conditions of puberty, pregnancy, menopause, and aging, and to environmental factors. The self-care limitations of the patient would arise from age or from lack of knowledge, skills, or essential resources.

Types of nursing cases with the life cycle focus include cases where the specific health focus is on (1) normal growth and development of infants, children, and youth, (2) the continuing psychological and social development of the adult, (3) pregnancy in girls, young women, and older women, and (4) the anatomical, physiological, and psychological changes of middle age and advanced age. The four general kinds of health care appropriate for the life cycle orientation would be adjusted to specific demands represented by the four types of nursing cases. The four types of cases require that a nurse have knowledge of growth and development as related to the phases in the life cycle; validated health care practices in the area of primary prevention; cultural practices related to infant or child care and to adolescent and adult life, family living, marital relations, and prepartum, intrapartum, and postpartum care; social and economic forces affecting the individual and family; and the influence of physical, biological, and social agents in the environment on individual, family, and community health. The life cycle focus, including its specific types of cases, is inherent in the health focus of the other five groups of cases. In a sense, it may be considered the core of any type of nursing situation.

Recovery

Recovery from disease, injury, or a functional disorder is the focus of health care. Medical treatment for the disease or injury has been instituted and has been effective in cure or regulation. Vital functions are stabilized. The characteristics of the medical therapy and its effects on the individual and the residual effects of the pathological process prescribe the needs for health care.

Specific cases within group 2 would be instances in which complete recovery is expected with no residual defect or disability, cases in which there will be a permanent structural or functional defect through loss of or defect in an organ or a part of the body, and cases in which a functional disorder is regulated by continuous therapy. Cases may also vary as to the degree of illness; there may be normal functioning, except for the affected structures or functions or degree of illness experienced. Health care needs would include:

1 Continued control of the recovery process through medical evaluation to determine the presence of sequelae and complications, the progress in recovery, and the effectiveness of disease regulation
2 Continued medical therapy and self-care specific for the cure or regulation of the disease, injury, or functional disorder and its effects
3 Specific protection when needed and possible in order to prevent sequelae and complications, defect, or disability resulting from the disease, injury, or functional disorder or from care measures
4 Early detection and medical diagnosis of complications with prompt treatment
5 Rehabilitation of the patient and the patient's self-image in the event of disfigurement, including loss of bodily parts or temporarily or permanently impaired functions
6 Health maintenance and promotion and specific protection from the actual or possible effects of the disease, injury, or functional disorder on general health and growth and development
7 Assistance to the patient and the family in assuming appropriate roles in health care, including self-care as related to the overall health care needs

In nursing cases of the group 2 type, therapeutic self-care would include care measures related to and derived from the disease process or functional disorder and measures derived from and related to medical diagnosis and therapy. Universal and developmental self-care requisites would require adjustments, not only to age and sex and environmental factors but also to the effects of the disease or injury and to the prescribed medical therapy. Self-care limitations may be caused by the effects of the disease process, the therapy used, the lack of necessary knowledge and skills, or a lack of resources.

Illness of Undetermined Origin

In group 3, health care is organized around signs and symptoms, degree of illness, and the need for medical diagnosis of the disease or disorder causing the signs and symptoms. A nursing case of this type is one in which the patient is suffering from a disorder with evident signs and symptoms and is either seriously ill and incapacitated, moderately or mildly ill, or functioning normally except for the presenting signs and symptoms of the disorder. The unknown causes of the signs and symptoms indicate that medical diagnosis and health evaluation is a principal health care need. The health care needs would include:

1 Prompt medical diagnosis of the nature, causes, and effects of the disease or disorder

2 Alleviation of symptoms through medical therapy and self-care measures with precautions for not masking symptoms

3 Prompt treatment and other protective care to prevent further structural or functional impairment or permanent defect and disability

4 Health maintenance and promotion required as a result of the nature of the signs and symptoms, the degree of illness, and actual or possible effects on the patient's general health

5 Assistance to the patient and the family in assuming appropriate roles in continuing health care, including self-care

The nursing aspects of group 3 situations would be similiar to group 2 situations. Participation in health evaluations and medical diagnostic measures could be a major component of self-care in group 3 situations, since the undetermined nature of the disorder would be a major concern of some patients that would affect both self-care and nursing.

Genetic and Developmental Defects and Biological Immaturity

The health focus is oriented to the care and treatment of patients with structural and functional defects or a state of immaturity present at birth. The defects may be hereditary or congenital. Immaturity may be a consequence of a premature birth or associated with low birth weight or other factors. Health care is oriented to making adjustments and adaptations necessitated by the defect or undeveloped state and to supplying the environmental conditions necessary to support life, facilitate integrated functioning, and contribute to present and future normalcy in daily living.

The characteristics of each structural or functional defect or behavioral disorder would determine how human functioning and daily living are impaired. For example, an infant with a cleft palate presents a different requirement for health care than does an infant with an inborn error in metabolism (in which certain biochemical reactions necessary for health and integrated functioning do not occur). Both the nature and extent of the effects of specific defects—for example, a cleft lip as compared with a cleft palate—on life, health, and effective living must be considered. Health care requirements in group 4 would include:

1 Continuous health care (including provision of a therapeutic environment) to achieve the adjustments and adaptations the patient needs for support of life processes and integrated functioning

2 Continuous health evaluation to determine the effects of the defect, behavioral disorder, or biological state on general health, growth, and development and functioning

3 Continuous diagnosis to determine the extent and the effects of the defect or disorder and the effects of therapy
4 Specific protection against complications or extension of present impairments into more disabling limitations
5 Rehabilitation of patient or parents of patient as indicated
6 Health maintenance and promotion and specific protection from actual or possible effects of the defect or disorder on general health, growth, and development and functioning
7 Assistance to the patient and family in assuming appropriate roles in continuing health care, including self-care

Nursing care is focused upon contributing to the necessary adaptations and adjustments required as a result of the defect or biological state and for maintaining essential environmental conditions. Rehabilitation may be of great importance in cases of this type. In some instances, major adjustments in family life are required. When defects are extensive and affect self-direction and behavioral control or mobility, provisions for continuing care within or outside the family setting are necessary.

Cure or Regulation

Health care in the form of active treatment for the cure or regulation of the effects of an injury, or disease, or functional disorder, including behavioral disorders not existent at birth, may be required during any period of a patient's life cycle. Major variations within this pattern relate to (1) the nature and extent of the injury and its effect, (2) the manner in which the disease or disorder manifests itself, including presenting signs and symptoms, (3) whether vital functions are stabilized or not stabilized, and (4) the degree of illness.

The following factors should be considered. Are the effects of the condition localized or generalized? Is the disease acute or chronic? If it is chronic, is it in an acute phase or in a phase of remission? Can the disease be cured? If it cannot, can it be regulated with continuous therapy? Is some degree of regulation possible when the disease process is progressive and cannot be cured or entirely controlled? Is palliative and symptomatic therapy required? Health care requirements would include:

1 Continuous care and medical therapy to cure or regulate the disease process or the functional disorder, to heal injured tissues, to alleviate symptoms, and to prevent disability
2 Therapy to stabilize or to protect vital functions and integrated functioning
3 Continuous control through evaluation of the progress of the disease process, the disorder, or the progress of recovery from the injury
4 Specific protection to prevent complications or the extension of

present effects of the disease, disorder, or injury that might result in disability

    5   Early diagnosis and prompt treatment of complications

    6   Health maintenance and promotion of general health, growth, and development

    7   Care to assist the patient in coping with suffering and disability when present

    8   Rehabilitation

    9   Assistance to the patient and family to assume appropriate roles in continuing health care, including self-care

The nursing aspects of the cure or regulation type of situation range from relatively simple to extremely complex. The specific symptoms, the degree of illness, the prognosis, the effects of the disease process on vital functions and integrated functioning, the amount and type of stress, as well as the form(s) of medical diagnosis and therapy and the effects of these measures, determine the kind and amount of self-care required by the patient. Self-care and nursing care are adjusted according to the changes in the patient's health state and to changes in medical diagnosis and therapy.

Stabilization of Integrated Functioning

In this type of case, health care is oriented to stabilization and control of the vital processes that have been disrupted by disease processes or by injury or to respiratory and cardiac functioning at birth. Variations in the individual case should be identified. What is the extent to which integrated functioning has been affected? Has an injury or its effects directly involved vital organs or affected integrated functioning? Is there immediate danger of death? Can any degree of control be established? If there is suffering, what is its nature and degree? Is the patient aware of the probable effects of the condition on life and health? Is there an anticipation of death or an uncontrolled fear of death? Whether the patient is an infant, child, adolescent, or adult is of great importance in nursing patients in this category. General health care requirements would include:

    1   Immediate institution of therapy to initiate or restore or stabilize and support vital functions and facilitate integrated functioning

    2   Continuous control through nursing observation and medical evaluation to determine the degree of functional deviation in the life processes and to adjust or institute therapy as required

    3   Nursing care and medical therapy to alleviate distressing symptoms and relieve suffering

    4   Nursing care and medical therapy to prevent complications, to diagnose them early, and to institute prompt treatment

5 Assistance to the ill or injured patient and family to sustain themselves in their suffering and to assume appropriate roles in the health situation

6 Care to enable a dying person and the family to face the reality of death

Terminal Illness

Health care is frequently oriented to the comfort and security of those who are in the terminal stages of illness. Care is directed to the control of persistent pain (if present) and to the regulation or control of other distressing symptoms (e.g., anorexia, dyspnea, frequency of urination, depression). Patients suffer increasing weakness and total distress.[7] Variations result from the natural history of the disorder, the types of symptoms being experienced, and the methods used for the regulation of symptoms. The aims of health care are to enable individuals with a terminal illness to live as themselves, to understand their illness and how to participate in care, to approach death in their own particular way, and to be with family, friends, and health care workers in an environment of security and trust. General health care requirements would include:

1 Effective medical management of the terminal illness
2 Active medical treatment as advisable
3 Continuous regulation of presenting sets of symptoms
4 Continuous effective meeting of the universal self-care requisites
5 Assistance directed to control of feelings of despair or rejection
6 Assistance to the patient and family to understand the patient's illness and its projected outcome and their roles in care and in preparation for the future
7 Continuing support to patient and family to enable them to sustain themselves and to have a measure of security

In situations of terminal illness, nurses ideally function with patients and family, physicians, paramedical personnel, and priests, ministers, or rabbis to institute and maintain a developmental environment for patients and all persons involved in their care.

HEALTH CARE SYSTEMS

Health care systems, including nursing systems, are constituted from actions deliberately selected and performed by individuals. Health care

[7]Cecily Saunders, *The Management of Terminal Illness,* Medical Publications, Ltd., London, 1967, p. 14.

systems include self-care and dependent-care systems created within the context of daily living. They also include care and service provided by ever-increasing numbers and types of health care personnel. People make health care systems; they are not naturally existent entities. The failure of nurses and others to recognize that health care systems must be made often results in inadequate communication with patients, families, and other health workers toward attaining the goal of coordination of human efforts.

Health care systems generated in part by physicians, nurses, and other health workers should be viewed as being constituted from the contributed actions of persons who have different social statuses and roles in social groups. Positions and roles in the field of health service indicate the kinds of actions that the persons filling them should be able to contribute to the formation of effective health care systems. What persons do contribute varies with their education, training, willingness to contribute, and other factors. The organizational charting of positions for a community health service, a hospital, or a nursing home is not necessarily a measure of the kind of health service being provided to consumers.

Nursing may be one of a number of health services needed by and provided to persons with health care requirements. The mix of health services being provided, the essential relationships among the services, and the individual and the combined contributions of the services to the health of an individual or a group constitute the health care system. From a service perspective, persons who seek and are provided with health care from institutionalized services have the *role of consumer and purchaser* of an available service. From the perspective of their relationship to the actual providers of care, they are in the *patient or client role*. In the role of consumer and purchaser people pay for what they receive through taxes, third party payments, or direct payment. In the role of patient or client, individuals should be helped to actively participate in their health care to the degree that their health and developmental states permit.

To provide nursing that is relevant to a patient's health care requirements, a nurse must be able to define his or her nursing role, including role relationships to the patient and to other health workers. Role definition requires awareness of the general dimensions of a patient's health care situation. It is a task that nurses perform at the time they enter health care situations and periodically thereafter. The seven groups of nursing situations organized according to differences in health care focuses and the general formulations of health care needs for each group (pages 136 to 145) can be used as an aid to the nurse's role definition.

Nurses require information to describe (1) the roles of the patient in each of the health services received (each service may be approached as a separate system or as a subsystem of the total health care system), (2) the contribution that each health service is capable of making to the patient's existing or projected health state, (3) the favorable or unfavorable effects of particular care measures on the patient, and (4) the way the various services must articulate when specific health care technologies are used or when specific results are sought. Further, since a patient may be affected favorably or unfavorably by any aspect of the health care situation or by the impact of the total system of health care, nurses as well as physicians must be alert not only to the effects of specific care measures on the patient but to the patient's level of tolerance for the health care system as a whole.

When the demands of using particular forms of health care on a patient become sufficiently burdensome, the patient may withdraw. Withdrawal may take a number of forms, for example, psychological withdrawal, as in depression or making the decision and taking action to remove oneself from the health care situation. Patients sign releases or simply walk away without informing health workers of their plans. Withdrawal may be evidence of the ineffectiveness or inefficiency of the system of health care.

Nurses seek information to describe why an individual has sought and received health care. Two questions are suggested as guides in securing information: (1) Why and from whom did the patient seek (is the patient seeking) health care? (2) Why and by whom was the patient accepted (is the patient being accepted) as a recipient of health care? The *subjective measures* of a person's need for health service include (1) state of satisfaction or dissatisfaction with his or her own structure and modes of functioning; (2) judgments about what is normal or abnormal, tolerable or intolerable; and (3) judgments about existing abilities to cope with the effects of perceived disorders of structure or functioning. Adults and older children have data on how they now appear, function, and feel to compare with their state at some previous time. In making these judgments, individuals use two sets of norms—what is usual or "normal" for them and norms of cultural deviation about what is "normal for the group," which may or may not be based on scientific knowledge.

Persons who seek health services may want help in order to find out what is "wrong" with them, to feel better, or to be cured. They may be seeking a health evaluation, assistance with a specific health problem, or the performance of some diagnostic or preventive health care measure such as vaccination. Health workers accept and take into account an individual's request and his or her evaluation of the need for health care as they engage in assessment of the health situation. The modes of delivery of health services to the people of a community will determine from whom health care is sought initially and who accepts individuals or groups for health care, thus affording them the position of patient in the health care system.

The *objective measure* of a person's need for health services of various types is either the overt presence of or some indication of disordered structure or functioning or evidence of a need for assistance in coping with a usual or unusual health care requirement. Assessment of health state or health care needs are health services that traditionally have been provided by physicians. Today, technologies for securing evidence to describe normality or abnormality of human structure and functioning are highly developed. These procedures are performed by a variety of health workers who have specialized preparation in the use of one or more of these technologies. For example, some public health nurses are prepared to test the hearing of individuals in the various age groups; when abnormalities are identified in individuals in the group tested, they are referred to the appropriate medical specialists.

Specific medical diagnostic procedures initiated by a physician may be preceded by a general health assessment. There is a developing trend for persons seeking health care in hospital outpatient departments or community health centers to have their needs for health care evaluated first by a physician's assistant or by a nurse. Nurses and physicians' assistants sometimes perform routine physical examinations. This initial objective assessment of health is not a substitute for the medical diagnostic process conducted by the physician or the detailed evaluation conducted by other specialists including nurses. When a nurse is the first health worker to see a person seeking or requiring health care, the nurse should attend to the patient's view of the need for care, to gross evidence of normality or abnormality of structure and functioning, and to what the individual indicates is the usual mode of functioning. The nurse may act at this time to meet the person's obvious needs for nursing assistance as well as to refer the person to a physician for care if this is indicated.

The initial seeking of subjective and objective information to measure a person's need for health care provides data to aid in formulating the purpose of the individualized health care system to be instituted for the patient. There may be a need at this time or later for cooperative action to resolve differences between the patient's subjective view of his or her needs and the objective views of the physicians, nurses, or other health workers. When the rights and responsibilities of individuals for their own health care are respected, each patient is permitted and encouraged to participate in the formulation of the purpose of the health care system to be produced and in the identification and clarification of roles. The purpose to which health care is directed serves to unify the efforts of physicians, nurses, and others who contribute to the patient's health care. If physicians and nurses and others do not communicate with the patient and among themselves, individuals in the health care situation may be working toward results that are not compatible with results being sought by other persons who are contributing to health care.

Seeking and analyzing data to aid in selecting constituent care elements for a system of health care that would be valid for the patient should be started when a person first seeks health care. It should be continued as long as the individual is under health care. This endeavor is necessary to provide persons seeking care with the care they need now as well as to foresee what they will need at some future time. Each health care facility (hospital, nursing home, clinic) that accepts a person or group as a recipient of service is responsible for the quality and amount of care provided. There should be established means for an initial and continued examination of the dimensions of each patient's health care situation in relation to the patient's view and health worker's view of reasons why health care is needed.

SELECTED READINGS

Butler, Robert N.: *Why Survive? Being Old in America*, Harper & Row, New York, 1975.

Citizens Board of Inquiry into Health Services for Americans: *Heal Yourself*, 2d ed., American Public Health Association, Washington, D.C., 1972.

Dubos, René: *Man Adapting*, Yale University Press, New Haven, 1967.

Galdston, Iago (ed.): *Beyond the Germ Theory: The Roles of Deprivation and Stress in Health and Disease*, New York Academy of Medicine, Health Education Council, New York, 1954.

Howard, Jan, and Anselm Strauss (eds.): *Humanizing Health Care*, Wiley, New York, 1975.

Hunt, Jennifer M., et al.: "Patients with Protracted Pain: A Survey Conducted at the London Hospital," *Journal of Medical Ethics*, vol. 3, 1977, pp. 61–73.

Knafl, Astin, and Helen K. Grace: *Families across the Life Cycle: Studies for Nursing*, Little, Brown, Boston, 1978.

Report of the Conference on Long-Term Health Care Data, Tucson, Arizona, May 12–16, 1975: *Medical Care*, vol. 14, May 1976, *Supplement*.

Saunders, Cecily: *The Management of Terminal Illness*, Hospital Medicine Publications, London, 1967. With an extensive bibliography.

Selye, Hans: *The Stress of Life*, McGraw-Hill, New York, 1956.

Shephard, David A. E.: "Principles and Practice of Palliative Care," *Canadian Medical Association Journal*, vol. 116, pp. 522–526.

Shipley, Roger R.: *The Health Experience*, Kendall/Hunt, Dubuque, Iowa, 1977. A textbook for college students.

Soane, Brendan: "The Literature of Medical Ethics: Bernard Häring," *Journal of Medical Ethics*, vol. 3, 1977, pp. 85–92.

Somers, Anne R., and Herman M. Somers: *Health and Health Care: Policies in Perspective*, Aspen Systems Corporation, Germantown, Md., 1977.

van Kaam, Adrian: *The Dynamics of Spiritual Self Direction*, Dimension Books, Denville, N.J., 1976.

Wilkes, E.: "Some Problems in Cancer Management," *Proceedings of the Royal Society of Medicine*, vol. 67, October 1974, pp. 1001–1005.

Variations
in Nursing Situations

COMPREHENDING THE DIMENSIONS
OF NURSING SITUATIONS

The number and variety of nursing situations are considerable. Nurses must establish the facts before they initiate nursing action. To do this, nurses *obtain, sort out,* and *interpret the meaning* of many types of information in order to have accurate and meaningful descriptions of nursing-relevant factors of health care situations. The factors of patient's age, health care focus and characteristic features of health care requirements, and interferences with deliberate action are useful indexes of the nursing requirements of patients because they reveal both the health and helping dimensions of nursing. These factors are interrelated, and to be of value they must be used as a set. The way in which these and other factors serve to reveal the nursing dimensions of health care situations and some of their interrelationships are described below.

A patient's *age* is an index of both the health and the helping dimensions of the nursing required. Human structure and functioning and health care needs vary with the periods of the human life cycle, from the prenatal period to old age. Health care requirements are thus specific for the various periods of the life cycle, though the basic requirements for life (universal self-care requisites) must be met during all periods. Age is an index of the amount and kind of assistance needed, since a person's powers for symbolization, thought, voluntary movement, and engagement in various kinds of deliberate action vary with the periods of the life cycle. Both the need for the use of health care and assisting technologies specific for a person's age group can be inferred from information about a patient's age. Individual differences must be recognized and taken into account.

When patients are in good to excellent states of health, age-relevant health care and assisting technologies may suffice. For example, health care of a newborn infant is related to adjustment to new environmental conditions, with emphasis on the prevention of disease. Because of newborn infants' helplessness, they must be cared for. However, if a person of any age is ill, disfigured, or disabled, or in a poor to fair state of health, health care technologies in addition to those required because of age will be needed. In these situations, assisting technologies will be selected in light of age and other factors that prevent or restrict a patient's engagement in deliberate action.

The characteristic features or the general nature of a patient's *requirement for health care* point out the *action that the patient or others must take* in the health care situation. As previously mentioned, age is an index of health care requirements specific to variations in human structure and functioning during the various stages of the life cycle. Poor health and the presence of disease, disfigurement, or disability establish other requirements for health care and indicate appropriate technologies of health care. The nature of the health results desired and the methods selected for achievement of the results would be indicators of the kinds of health workers required and their roles and of the patient's roles in the achievement of health results. Information about the patient's age, state of health and disease, the reasons the patient sought or was accepted for health care, and knowledge of valid health care technologies are necessary if nurses are to comprehend quickly and accurately the health care focus and the general features of a patient's requirements for health care. These requirements would indicate the dimensions of therapeutic self-care needed by the patient on a continuous or periodic basis. They would also guide the nurse in identifying and describing obstacles to the patient's engagement in self-care.

Interferences with a patient's *engagement in deliberate action* point out (1) the general dimensions of the nurse's responsibility for a patient, (2) the methods that can be validly used in assisting a patient, (3) the probable duration of a patient's need for assistance, and (4) the patient's future potential as a self-care agent. Interferences with deliberate action, as previously indicated, are related to age as well as to health state and to the kind of health care required. Information in regard to all types of interferences must be obtained. The general features of each specific interference must be known if the nurse is to use the information in making inferences about the four enumerated dimensions of assistance. Since interferences with a person's engagement in deliberate action set up requirements for health care (for example, rehabilitation in the event of disability), interferences are indexes of both the helping and health dimensions of nursing.

Individuals who can benefit from nursing may be of any age and any state of development and health. When multiperson units such as families become the subject of care and service from nurses, the constituent members of the unit may be of similar or dissimilar ages and states of development and health. Nurses' descriptions of persons who are seeking or under nursing care must take into consideration age, developmental state, and health state. If these three factors are not investigated and characterizing data are not obtained, nurses will not have an adequate basis for understanding the helping and health aspects of nursing, since they influence both aspects of nursing. Age as a factor in the production of variety in nursing situations will be discussed. The influences of age and other factors on the production of variations in the therapeutic self-care demands and the self-care agency of patients will then be addressed.

AGE AS A FACTOR IN NURSING

Age of the patient is an important factor in every nursing situation. It normally is closely related to the characteristics of a person's behavior, and it has meaning in relationship to the self-care behavior of the patient and the nursing behavior of the nurse. Age also has a number of meanings in a given society, and these meanings have a variety of influences on the lives of the members of that society. Nurses must be aware of these meanings and their influences, since such knowledge is related to the consideration of age in every nursing situation.

The Meaning of Age

Age is most frequently thought of in terms of chronological age, the period of time between birth and succeeding time periods. Chronological age is measured in seconds, minutes, hours, days, weeks, months, and years. Nurses may care for infants whose age can be measured in seconds as well as for persons who age can be measured in decades. In prenatal life, chronological age is measured in time intervals within the nine-month gestation period (the first, second, and third trimesters). A person may be an adult chronologically but be retarded physically, intellectually, or behaviorally. Aging is associated with physical changes that may affect the usual integrated functioning of the adult.

Developmental age refers to the combinations of qualities, powers, and capacities that develop naturally in each person in light of hereditary factors and environmental conditions (for example, appearance, language, posture, and locomotion). The developmental age of an individual is determined by identifying physical and behavioral developments and comparing them with chronological age group norms. Characteristic growth and developmental pictures of individuals by chronological age periods are valuable guides to nurses in understanding health care requirements (including care to promote normal growth and development) and limitations for deliberate action. Each nurse must be constantly alert to advances in the knowledge of human growth and development and in technologies that foster normal growth, development, and health by age group.

Growth in physical size is readily observable and measurable. Since individuals grow at different rates, children of the same chronological age may vary in physical size. Persons who are small or large because of hereditary factors or whose natural growth has been retarded in some way, such as through malnutrition, may have problems in accepting themselves and in being accepted by others. Problems may also arise from a child's degree of development or maturity, which determines what a child can do at a particular age. If development is slow, help may be needed in allaying the child's fears that he or she will not be normal or be able to do what other children of the same age can do. If the rate of maturing is rapid, the child may need guidance in accepting himself or herself and relating to other children.[1]

Some societies establish the chronological age at which individuals, according to law, are capable of making certain decisions, of entering into contracts, and of being held legally responsible for their acts. In the United States, this age is part of either the common law of the country or the civil law of the states. According to common law, for example, the *age of majority* or adulthood is 21 years for both men and women. In some states, however, it is 18 years for women. Before a person reaches the legal age of adulthood, the law recognizes other ages such as the age of discretion, the age of consent, and military age. The *age of discretion* means that a minor at the age of 14 years is recognized as possessing sufficient knowledge to be responsible for certain acts and to exercise certain powers. A minor under 7 years of age is conclusively presumed incapable of criminal intent, and a minor between the ages of 7 and 14 years is considered incapable of criminal intent unless there is proof to

[1]Dorothy V. Whipple, *Dynamics of Development: Euthenic Pediatrics,* McGraw-Hill, New York, 1966. See Chap. 41, "Age-Portrait Summaries," pp. 592–615, for concise descriptions relevant to health care.

the contrary. The *age of consent*, which varies by state, is the age at which a person is recognized as legally competent to consent to marriage and to other acts.

Laws also protect persons who have not reached adult status. These laws hold natural and adoptive parents legally responsible for the support of a child. Support includes the provision of food, clothing, shelter, education, and health care. Legally, parents are responsible for the protection of the health and well-being of their child, including the development of character and personal and social values.

A person's chronological age and sex relate to status within a family, for example, the status and roles of husband and wife, mother and father, son and daughter, and brother and sister. Status and role define the duties and responsibilities of the individual toward other members of his or her family.

Age as it is discussed here is a relatively important factor in cultural practices related to infant and child care and supervision, instruction of children in self-care and sex attitudes, education toward independence, teaching skills and beliefs, formal education, care of the aged, marriage, and the family. The respect and care given to the young, to the elderly, and to women during pregnancy and the assistance given to individuals in the transitional period from youth to adulthood all reflect how a society views the importance of these age-related events. A patient's attitude or the attitude of family members and the attitude of the nurse in these areas are important influences in each nursing situation.

The Influence of Age on Nursing

The chronological and developmental ages of a patient affect the health and helping dimensions of the nursing situation in a number of ways. They influence (1) the social relations of nurse and patient, (2) techniques for assisting, communicating, and socializing to roles, (3) appropriate nurse responses to a patient's behavior, (4) the frequency and duration of the contacts between nurse and patient, (5) the scope of the nurse's responsibility for protecting the patient as a person, (6) the nurse's relationship to members of the patient's family, and (7) the health and self-care needs of the patient. Understanding these influences requires a comprehensive fund of knowledge of human growth and development, social networks, and cultural practices as well as knowledge of communication and social interaction theories and technologies. This knowledge must be applied in collecting descriptive information about patients, interpreting the information, and using it in designing and providing nursing assistance for adults and children.

Nurses and nursing students may be in the adolescent stage of the life cycle, which is preparatory for access to specialized work in the society. They may also be adults preparing for or engaging in specialized work. Their patients may be of any age. Ideally, the nurse's behavior should convey acceptance and respect toward all patients. This is, of course, mature behavior and requires that the nurse recognize each patient as a person, as a member of a family, and as one who has a unique heredity and life history. Mature behavior in interpersonal situations also demands from the nurse an awareness of the need for adjusting his or her behavior to practices in the patient's culture that regulate social relations by age and position in the family or community.

Providing nursing to a child differs in several ways from providing nursing to an adult. The age status of a patient as an adult, a neonate, an infant, a child, or a youth has important implications for nursing regardless of the patient's state of health and disease. The adult's right and responsibility to make decisions is recognized by society, as is the child's inability to do this. The developed and developing powers of the child must be identified and fostered within the nursing situation. Nurses should be acutely aware of the limits for realistic behavioral expectations for children according to age. Nurses should also provide for differences in environmental needs and be alert to signals of health problems by age groups. Evidence of failure to grow and develop as well as evidence of regressive changes and dysfunction by age group must be understood by nurses.

Nurses should understand the quality of trust, including its importance in effective interpersonal relations and in human growth and development. The trust a patient has in a nurse, the nurse's acceptance of it, and the nurse's respect for the patient are interacting forces that aid in the maintenance of the nurse-patient relationship. The nurse at times will be required to set limits for the behavior of children, youth, and sometimes adults as it relates to the patient's or the nurse's well-being. When trust, acceptance, and respect prevail, limit setting is more likely to be viewed as help given and not as restraint or coercion.

Age-Specific Factors in Nursing Children

In nursing situations involving infants, children, and youth, the patient continues in his or her role of *a dependent who must be cared for or guided by a responsible adult*. Nursing of young patients is a mix of care measures, which each patient needs because of his or her (1) chronological and developmental age, (2) genetic heritage, (3) unique personality, (4) physical and social environment, and (5) health state and related health care needs. Nursing in situations where the patient is young may involve direct care of the patient by the nurse and assistance to parents or guardians in learning to give the continuous care needed by the child or to cooperate with health workers. The nurse's dual relationship to child and to parents makes the nurse role complex and requires that techniques of assisting be adapted to the needs of the child and the needs of the parents, who may be adolescents or adults.

In the direct nursing care of a young patient, the nurse selects ways of assisting that are in accord with the patient's age and stage of growth and development. *Caring for, acting or doing for,* and *providing an environment that promotes development* are valid ways for nursing infants and young children. *Guiding* and *supporting* the child in self-care action are appropriate methods of nursing older children to the degree permitted by the health state. Older children and adolescents can learn and want to be responsible for their personal health-related care. They will also want and need guidance and supervision from a responsible adult, though at times they will resist these efforts. Sustained interest of the nurse in the health care efforts of the young patient can make a great contribution toward the patient's becoming an effective self-care agent. Nurses should endeavor to help adolescents develop beneficial self-care practices. When nurses know the adult family members have incorporated practices harmful to health into their daily living, guidance of youth toward physical and mental health should be an important nursing concern.

When children have continuing therapeutic self-care needs that the parents are incapable of meeting, care responsibilities for the child may be distributed between the nurse and the parents. The distribution should be based on an objective consideration of the parent's limitations for giving the needed therapeutic care. When infants and sick children are placed in hospitals or other health care institutions, parents should be permitted to be with the child and fulfill some of the care responsibilities for the child whenever possible and prudent.

When parents cannot be with their child, the child should have a person to whom he or she can relate during various periods of the day. In an institutional situation, this role may be assigned to a person trained in child care rather than in nursing. This practice is appropriate when most of the care needs of the infant or child are not of the specialized type of care required as a result of disease, injury, or defect. Nurses should be able to give both aspects of care to children, but they also should be able to work cooperatively with both parents and with persons trained for child care. In long-term care institutions or when children are ill at home for prolonged periods, their formal education should be continued under the direction of qualified teachers.

The nature of the interpersonal relationship between a nurse and an infant, child, or adolescent patient is of paramount importance. It should communicate trust. The young patient should be able to feel that the nurse is a responsible adult who is interested in him or her and to whom he or she can turn for help. The nurse fosters the child's growth and development and at the same time contributes to the achievement of other specific health results. It is thus essential that the nurse know about the present developmental state of the child and how children develop cognitively and use knowledge at various ages.

The relationships between the nurse and the mother, father, or guardian of a child also may be affected by the age of the nurse or of the parents as well as by cultural factors. In cases where the parents have differing opinions about the care needs of the child, the nurse may find it necessary to work with both parents for the child's well-being. This situation is a complex one. Some nurses may not be sufficiently competent to cope with it.

A nursing situation in which the patient is an infant, child, or youth continues as long as the patient requires specialized therapeutic care or until the parents or guardians have overcome their limitations for giving the needed care or assistance. Nurses should select methods that will benefit both the child and the parents. For example, if an infant or child has to be fed using a technique adapted for a cleft lip or palate, it may be appropriate for the nurse to involve the parents early in learning to feed the infant. Parents may need periodic guidance and supervision from a nurse when they are giving and managing the continuous therapeutic care required by a sick or disabled child or when they are giving therapeutic care to a well child.

When a child's integrated functioning is seriously disturbed or the health care technologies are complex and interrelated and in situations where the child's suffering is intense, nurses should not involve the parents in the technical aspects of the child's health care. In situations where parents must become technically able to participate in or completely provide the continuous health care for their child at home, nurses must carefully determine how the parents can be assisted without harm to them or to the child. In situations where children have birth defects or an illness that places parents in an adverse light with or without reason, or when children are unwanted and rejected, parents may need health care for their own sake as well as for that of the child.

In infant, child, or adolescent nursing situations, there should be an open line of communication between nurse(s) and parents and nurse(s) and physician(s). This is necessary because of the legal status of the patient as a minor and the patient's limitations in understanding and decision making. Because children are immature emotionally and physically, they cannot be expected to be responsible agents in their own health care or in coordination of the various parts of care. The role of the adolescent in self-care, including its coordination with other aspects of health care, may be extended with guidance and supervision. The nurse must be aware of prescribed roles, rights, and responsibilities. Parents sometimes may not be in contact with adolescent sons or daughters or assume responsibility for their care or support. Guidance and support from interested and accepting adults are essential to meet developmental needs of young people who have taken on or are about to take on the duties of adult members of a society.

In caring for a minor, physicians must be in direct communication with the child's parents and nurses. The physician has an ethical and legal responsibility to keep parents informed of the child's health state. Some physicians also accept responsibility for guiding parents in fostering the growth and development of the child. A failure in communication between a child's parents and the physician may have adverse effects on the total health care situation, including the nursing component.

In some child nursing situations, it is essential that the child's nurse talk with nurses in another agency in coordinating the care of a child. A nurse giving care to a child at home, for example, may want to discuss nursing information with a nurse in an outpatient clinic or in a hospital before a clinic visit or hospitalization. Nurses, too, may find it necessary to contact the child's teachers or assist the child's parents in doing this whenever the child's daily health care needs must be given attention at school. When two or more health care agencies are involved in providing health services, coordination of their activities is important for the effective health care of both children and adults. Channels of communication should be provided and kept open to facilitate interagency coordination of health care for individual patients.

Age-Specific Factors in Nursing Adults

From the viewpoint of the patient's age, adult nursing situations differ from child situations in that adults have the right to decide about the kinds of health care they will accept and the responsibility to act for themselves in matters of self-care and health. Adults may be emotionally or socially dependent on other people as a result of inadequate physical or personality development or because of the effects of disease, injury, or disability. However, they are not dependent in the way children are because of their age.

In child nursing situations, the child's age is a signal to the nurse of how to care for and communicate with the child, of growth and developmental needs, and of needs to control regression stimulated by illness or by environmental factors. The adult patient's age is a signal to the nurse that the patient is responsible for himself or herself and his or her dependents (unless the patient is incompetent from developmental or other defects). A patient's age tells the nurse that the patient is able to communicate as an adult but at a level that is influenced by habits of perceiving and thinking and that needs for help in self-care arise from health state or health care requirements. Adult age also may point to needs for assistance in accepting and living in a state of social dependency resulting from illness or treatment, in becoming self-directing about matters of self-care, and in learning to seek and use nursing services including guidance and consultation in self-care.

In adult nursing situations, a nurse-family relationship may or may not exist. When an adult patient is not physically or mentally competent to manage his or her own affairs or make decisions about health care, nurses may have frequent contacts with a responsible member of the patient's family. When family members in a home provide the continuous care needed by a patient, nurses may instruct, supervise, and consult with family members.

Sometimes adult patients who are incompetent have legally appointed guardians. Adult patients who may be seriously ill or aged may give another responsible adult the power of attorney to transact business for them in accordance with regulations established by law. If adults are unable to decide or act for themselves, a family member, preferably the closest relative, should act for them. Adult children often care for their aged parents, or a wife may care for a seriously ill husband. When an adult has a legally appointed guardian, the guardian occupies much the same position as the natural parents of a child.

Other age-related considerations are of great importance in nursing situations. Adult patients who are aware of their experiences and of the events that occur in the health care situation serve as information and communication centers in the health care situation. They interact with health workers, other persons who provide services, and family members and friends. The frequency and duration of contacts, the variety of social contacts, the content of communications, and a patient's interpretation of and reactions to his or her experiences are influencing factors on health care and nursing. Health workers place demands on patients to make observations, to reveal information, and, at times, to give messages to other health workers and to manage their own care. It is important that adult patients be helped to become responsible agents in their own health care. It is also important that nurses and other health workers not burden a patient with their own coordinating duties.

The nursing situation may also be affected by an adult's social responsibilities. The adult patient's health and health care may interfere with family life, work, and other aspects of adult living. The adult may be unable to finance health care, care for dependent children, or provide for family needs. An adult patient's motivation to overcome or compensate for limitations resulting from injury or disability may be greatly influenced by family and work responsibilities.

VARIATIONS IN THERAPEUTIC SELF-CARE DEMANDS

A therapeutic self-care demand has been described as a prescription for the self-care measures to be performed in order to meet identified sets of self-care requisites—universal, developmental, and health-deviation (Chapter 3). A person's therapeutic self-care demand is one of the two patient variables of nursing systems, the other being the patient's ability to engage in self-care, that is, self-care agency. A person's therapeutic self-care demand varies with age, developmental state, health state, and other factors.

Variations in therapeutic self-care demands of members of a nursing population and variations in the demands of individuals from time to time may be identified and described in terms of (1) the particular values of each one of the universal self-care requisites, (2) the particular values of the two kinds of developmental requisites, and (3) the presence of health-deviation self-care requisites and their derivation, for example, from a pathological process, or as medically prescribed and associated with medical diagnoses or treatment measures, or as associated with regulation of the effects of medical diagnostic and treatment measures. Given particular values of specific self-care requisites, variations in therapeutic self-care demands may result from the methods selected for meeting them and from the measures of care (action systems) necessary for using a method in meeting a requisite.

Two possible variations in the mix of self-care requisites exist: (1) a combination of universal and developmental requisites and (2) a combination of universal, developmental, and health-deviation requisites. The eight types of nursing situations classified by health care focus (Chapter 6) suggest these two variations. Whenever the life cycle focus prevails, there is a mix of universal and developmental requisites. For example, in the event of mental retardation or other forms of retarded development with the absence of injury or overt disease processes, there would be a need for adjustments in the values of the universal and developmental requisites and for the use of appropriate methods for meeting them, for example, the selection and use of appropriate instructional methods and educational experiences and the appropriate regulation of living conditions to foster the retarded child's personal development, including involvement in self-care.

In the remaining seven types of nursing situations health-deviation requisites are present in addition to universal and developmental requisites. These seven types of nursing situations also vary according to (1) the number and kinds of health-deviation requisites and the relationships among these requisites and (2) the degree to which the normal values and ways of meeting the universal and developmental requisites are changed.

For example, when persons have the condition that has the medical name of *chronic congestive heart failure,* the patient's health care focus, if it is therapeutic, is on self-management and meeting specific self-care requisites directed toward the regulation of the burden on the heart and toward the prevention of complicating conditions. Under the care of physicians and nurses and with assistance from family members, patients:

1 Remain on a prescribed amount of bed rest
2 Maintain a posture that prevents dyspnea
3 Engage in some exercise, avoiding exertion that results in dyspnea
4 Take precautions against contracting infections
5 Act to regulate stress-producing conditions
6 Control sodium chloride intake and use prescribed medications to regulate excretion of body fluids; monitor for effects and results
7 Use prescribed medications to regulate cardiac functioning; monitor for effects and results
8 Monitor for known complications and general sense of well-being or illness

This set of health-deviation self-care requisites includes ones that are essentially adjustments in the universal self-care requisites. The regulatory contribution to a person's well-being made by meeting each health-deviation self-care requisite and the interrelationships among the requisites must be understood by nurses if they are to help patients in managing themselves and in understanding and meeting their therapeutic self-care demands.

Nurses should have knowledge about recurring disorders of human structure and functioning, including knowledge of their natural history, in order to understand the associated health-deviation self-care requisites. This knowledge includes how the values of some or all of the universal self-care requisites may be affected. Specific pathological processes usually affect the values of some but not all of the universals. When a disease becomes generalized (e.g., cancer) or when a person is critically ill, nurses must operate with continuing awareness that all of the universal self-care requisites may require continuing adjustment.

Variations in therapeutic self-care demands of individuals also result from the presence of factors that affect the choice of methods for meeting universal self-care requirements (and other requisites). Age, sex, states of development and health, and personal interests and concerns give rise to such factors. Methods selected for meeting each universal self-care requisite must be adjusted to certain conditions; for example, in maintaining a sufficient intake of food, the condition of being an infant or a child requires the use of methods that are effective for feeding infants or young children. A selected method must be able to surmount interfering factors, as in feeding by gavage when a person of any age cannot swallow.

Factors in addition to age and degree of physical maturation that condition the methods of meeting each universal self-care requisite and the degree to which each can be met should be understood by nurses. Identification of such factors is a necessary step in the calculation of the therapeutic self-care demands of individuals. Survey lists that identify factors affecting the choice of methods for meeting each of the eight universal self-care requisites should be helpful tools in nursing practice. In 1977, the author, in collaboration with Janet L. Fitzwater, developed eight tentative survey lists as a part of an exploration of problems associated with the continuous and effective meeting of the universal self-care requisites of patients in one long-term care institution. The survey list of factors that affect the meeting of the requisites for maintaining adequate intakes of water and food is reproduced in Table 7-1. When nurses identify that one or some combination of these factors is operative in a patient, a next step is to determine methods that will work in meeting the self-care requisite. Sometimes medical collaboration and medical prescriptions will be required.

Table 7-1 Survey List of Factors Affecting Choice of Care Methods

Set One

1 Diminished appetite or aversion to food (anorexia)
2 Reluctance or refusal to eat or drink water or fluids
3 Unable to eat or drink because of loss of awareness

Set Two

4 Nausea
5 Vomiting

Set Three

6 Interferences with control of the tongue and muscles of mastication
7 Dysphagia

Set Four

8 Changes in the mouth, pharynx, esophagus, stomach or bowels that affect the intake, mastication, movement, digestion, and absorption of food

Set Five

9 Available water, fluids, and foods
   a Displeasing to sight or taste or smell
   b Not in a state compatible with powers of mastication and deglutition
   c Not in accord with cultural prescriptions
   d Do not meet prescriptions for qualitative or quantitative sufficiency
10 Water, fluids, and food not available
   a When desired
   b When needed

Nurses' use of such survey lists is essential in nursing situations where patients are under nursing care for prolonged periods of time or in any nursing situation where the nurse bears the full responsibility for calculating and meeting patients' therapeutic self-care demands. Without the use of such lists for data-gathering purposes, nurses may fail to adequately attend to the meeting of patients' universal self-care requisites. Such failures on the part of nurses (or dependent-care agents) may result in the illness, disability, or death of patients.

VARIATIONS IN SELF-CARE AGENCY

In nursing practice, the capability of patients to engage in self-care can be assessed according to three scales—developmental, operational, and adequacy.[2] In taking this type of diagnostic approach to making judgments about the self-care agency of patients, nurses seek to determine the following with respect to self-care:

1 What individuals have learned to do and do consistently
2 What individuals *can and cannot do* now or in the future because of existing or predicted conditions and circumstances
3 Whether what individuals have *learned to do* and *can now do* is equal to meeting all the current or projected demands on them to engage in self-care, that is, to meeting their therapeutic self-care demands now or at some future time

Since self-care is learned behavior, nurses must take into account the readiness and the capabilities of individuals for extending or deepening their abilities to engage in self-care.

Variations in the self-care agency of patients can thus be understood and examined in relation to:

1 Self-care measures that patients know how to and usually do perform (repertoire of self-care practices; usual components of the self-care system)
2 Action limitations that restrict the performance of what patients know how to do with respect to self-care (limitations that interfere with the performance of the operations required for the decision-making and productive phases of self-care)
3 Self-care measures to be performed in order to meet known self-care requisites for which patients have or do not have requisite knowledge, skill, or willingness (adequacy or limitation of knowledge, skills and tech-

[2]Nursing Development Conference Group, *Concept Formalization in Nursing: Process and Product,* 2d ed., Little, Brown, Boston, 1979. Chap. 8, "Self-Care Agency—Diagnostic Considerations," Fig. 8-1.

, niques, or willingness to meet known self-care requisites using particular care methods)

4 Patients' potential for extending or deepening their knowledge of self-care and mastering the techniques necessary to perform required self-care measures that are not within their existing self-care repertoires (potential for further developments to extend or deepen self-care agency)

5 Patients' potential for consistent and effective performance of new and essential self-care measures, including the integration of essential self-care measures into the self-care system and daily life

To accumulate and validate knowledge about variations in the self-care agency of nursing populations, it would seem practical to approach the five possible variations separately. In particular nursing situations, nurses should consistently investigate the first three variations. If there is a lack of adequacy (third variation), the fourth and fifth variations, dealing with patient potential, should be investigated.

The five variations in self-care agency are judged to be relatively exhaustive. They should be good organizers for the purposes of nursing practice and research. Nurses can use these variations (or the descriptive phrases in parentheses) to formulate judgments about the self-care agency of patients. When these judgments are based on enough empirical evidence, they are in the nature of nursing diagnoses. To complete these judgments as nursing diagnoses, nurses need to identify and describe the factors that have conditioned or are now conditioning the particular variation. For example, if the self-care repertoire of an individual is more extensive than that of family members or the culture group to which the individual belongs, it may be important for a nurse to know the factors associated with this difference. Knowing the value of self-care agency in the five variations is necessary in nursing situations. If nurses do not know the factors associated with these values, they will not have an adequate base for helping the patient with the regulation of the exercise or development of self-care agency.[3]

THE PATIENT'S HEALTH STATE

Well-being and illness are critical factors in nursing situations, for they are the determinants of the appropriate health care focus and the types of health results sought. Nurses must have information about the general health states of patients as well as information about conditions and events associated with the specific diseases from which patients suffer.

Information about the patient's health state is obtained from a number of sources: the patient, persons who live with the patient, the patient's

[3]Ibid., Chap. 7, "Self-Care Agency: A Conceptual Analysis," Fig. 8-2.

physician, the medical history, and the recorded results of physical and other examinations and laboratory tests. Understanding the meaning of such information requires that nurses have knowledge of normal integrated human functioning, pathological conditions, basic procedures of health evaluation, and the purposes of medical diagnosis and therapy in relation to health and disease. Nurses, in making observations of patients or of records and reports on patients, initially and continuously determine evidence that will enable them to understand patients' health states.

Specifically, the information the nurse seeks will include descriptions of (1) the degree of illness, its causes, and whether it is acute or chronic; (2) obvious injuries or defects; (3) the patient's present behavior patterns (what he or she does or does not do); (4) the effects of disease or disordered function being experienced by the patient (including pain, alterations of body temperature, alterations of respiratory and circulatory functioning, gastrointestinal functioning, genitourinary functioning, nervous and musculoskeletal functioning, alterations of the skin and its appendages, and bleeding and anemia), and (5) possible or known effects of the patient's present health state on integrated functioning and effective living.

It is important that nurses know if the disease or disorder the patient has is one of the common causes of death. Vascular diseases of the central nervous system, acute coronary disease, other heart diseases, and malignancy are leading causes of death. The effect a disease may have upon the life of a patient is a factor that affects the outlook and behavior of the patient and family as well as that of the nurse. The effects of a patient's illness upon the family is very important in all nursing situations.

The physician's view of the patient's health situation is reflected in the medical diagnosis and prognosis, the recorded medical history, and the results of the physical examinations and laboratory tests. The kind of therapy the physician prescribes and the diagnostic and other measures the physician uses are also significant for nursing diagnosis.

In nursing situations where patients are under active medical care there is need for discussion between the patient's nurse(s) and the physician so that the nurse can determine (1) how the physician views the patient's health situation, (2) the aspects of the patient's medical care regimen that should become parts of the patient's self-care system on a long-term or short-term basis, including monitoring of selected aspects of human functioning, (3) which physician, if there is more than one, has the position of responsibility for integrating and coordinating the patient's medical care, and (4) the projected duration of active medical care for the patient. It is only through the conscious and deliberate efforts of physicians and nurses to communicate with each other about the daily care of the patient that nursing care and medical care can be coordinated to produce an effective health care system for the patient.

During the initial period of nursing diagnosis, a patient may be rel-atively healthy; slightly, moderately, or seriously ill; injured; or suffering from defect or disability. Life experiences, present environmental situa-tion, and interests and concerns will influence the patient's view of the health state and the need for health care as well as the patient's readiness or ability to cooperate with health care workers.[4] A patient's view of his or her health situation may be related to the characteristics of the disease process itself. There is a process of becoming ill. There are also modes of adaptation to illness and to the recovery process. The disease, the kinds of symptoms, and the rapidity with which they develop help to describe the process of becoming ill. One physician who studied patients who had cerebral vascular accidents or strokes described the patients as having been plunged within a relatively short time into "a rather unfamiliar and complicated life situation" that "is rapidly changing," a situation where the "full import and meaning cannot be readily grasped in the initial states."

In describing their experiences and reactions in the initial phases of the disease process, the patients' responses demonstrated (1) personality resources—for example, "courage, self-control, patience, and accep-tance," (2) minimization and rationalization of initial symptoms, (3) res-ignation to the outcome of the illness, and (4) "mounting apprehensiveness and heightened dependency." In strokes, as in other illnesses where there can be extensive brain damage, there may be unawareness of illness or of deficits such as that resulting from a paralysis. The stroke patient's view of his or her illness during its early phases and the tendency to maximize or minimize difficulties rather than to see them realistically were indicators of reactions in later phases of the illness and in the recovery process.[5]

In studying diseases and patterns of illness it is important for nurses and nursing students to learn what has been presently identified about patterns of adaptation. In studies of two types of disabling illness, the following patterns were noted: (1) insightful acceptance, (2) a struggle with conflicts brought on by disability through projection and other psy-chological mechanisms, (3) exaggeration of dependency and the demand-ing of more help than might actually be required, and (4) a slowly developing depression with loss of motor ability, a sense of failure in coping with events with resultant sadness, and feelings of helplessness that may be unrecognized by the patient initially. Once they are recog-nized, however, they are not denied.[6]

[4] Andie L. Knutson, *The Individual, Society, and Health Behavior*, Russell Sage Foun-dation, New York, 1969, pp. 180–193.
[5] Montague Ullman, "Health Deviations and Behavior," in Dorothea E. Orem and Kitty S. Parker (eds.), *Nursing Content in Preservice Nursing Curriculum*, Catholic Uni-versity of America Press, Washington, D.C., 1964, pp. 74–76.
[6] Ibid., pp. 78–80.

Patients' views of their health situation influence their own roles and nurses' roles in the nursing situation. What responsibility can the patient bear now and fulfill effectively in the future? In light of the patients' perception of and responses to their health situation, what kind of assistance is required to identify the patient role? How can patients be helped to face and accept the demands that illness or injury place upon them? Nurses, especially those who have not experienced personal or family problems of a serious nature or who have not been victims of a natural disaster, may not be perceptive about the impact of personal loss or of excessive physical and emotional demands upon the individual.

Illness and injury generally impose hardships upon people. The outcome of illness and injury may be uncertain; a person is faced with the unknown and may experience anxiety, fear of permanent disability, lifelong suffering, or even death. In some instances patients must make decisions about the kinds of measures they will permit the physician to use. Nurses should be able to envision the meaning that illness or disability and being a patient have for individuals.

If a nurse sees only movements toward health, toward more effective living, without seeing the demands and burdens that injury, illness, and health care place upon a patient, the basis for nursing diagnosis and prescription is incomplete. The nursing perspective will be inaccurate, and the nurse will not have a sound basis for proceeding toward the nursing goal of assisting the patient in responsible action in matters of self-care. The patient may be willing to accept care given by the nurse, may demand care from the nurse, or may be disinterested in or even refuse care. Patients may need help in understanding not only the self-care demands on them but also the rationale for particular self-care requisites or for sets of requisites. A nurse's diagnostic investigations may reveal that a first task is to help the individual learn how to cooperate in the determination of needs that can be met through nursing.

Health Results

Nurses' investigations of and judgments about the self-care requisites of patients take into consideration the reasons why patients are under health care and the health results to be achieved. The types of health results mentioned previously include the maintenance and promotion of health, including the prevention of disease, defect, and disability; the cure or regulation of disease processes; the preservation of life through the initiation, preservation, or restoration of vital processes; rehabilitation toward effective living in the event of disability; and being able to live and function with some degree of ease and personal satisfaction during a terminal illness.

When patients with health disorders are under nursing care, nurses must have or seek authoritative information about the natural history of the specific disease processes. The medical literature or physician and nurse specialists with extensive experience in caring for patients with particular diseases are sources. Such knowledge enables nurses to envision the kinds of health results associated with the disease. For example, through fact-gathering activities, the nurse finds that a patient has been diagnosed as having a stone in the right ureter. From observations of the patient and from the physician's notes, the nurse is aware that the pain is severe and the patient is in great distress. The nurse draws upon knowledge from anatomy, physiology, and pathology in forming a mental picture of what is presently in process in the patient. The nurse understands the physiological problem resulting from the presence of the stone and the mechanics related to the possible passage of the stone, considering the size and shape of the stone in relation to the diameter of the ureter and to its tissue structure and physiology. Causes of stone formation and of preventive measures come to mind. The nurse draws upon his or her knowledge of pain and of physiology, psychology, and pathology in making observations and judgments.

From reading the physician's medical orders for the patient and from talking with the physician, the nurse also becomes aware that the physician does not plan at this time to use surgical techniques to remove the stone but will first see if the patient can pass the stone, using drug therapy as indicated. The nurse becomes aware that the patient will be enduring the painful process of passing the stone, with all its distressing effects, and concludes that the desired, immediate health-related results needed by the patient are four in number: (1) the elimination of the stone, (2) prevention or control of complications, (3) relief from pain, and (4) reduction of physical and psychological stress. The nurse knows the distressing effects produced by the passing of stones and is aware of the results to be sought and the kinds of care measures that will be effective while the patient lives through the process of passing the stone. Nurses' knowledge of health, disease, and medical diagnostic and therapeutic modalities should include their points of articulation with nursing. The patient variables, therapeutic self-care demand and self-care agency, provide appropriate linkages.

PLACE AS A FACTOR IN NURSING

The place in which a patient is given nursing care is a variable that requires consideration in nursing situations. Place is of importance for several reasons. Some of the reasons can be best expressed as questions. Is the patient away from his or her usual place of residence and from an accustomed environmental setting? If so, what is the patient's outlook? Is the experience stress-producing, accepted, or even comforting to the patient? A patient's response to being a patient in a hospital, an extended care facility, a nursing home, a community health center, a clinic, or an outpatient department of a hospital is influenced by his or her knowledge and attitudes regarding health care.

Although they provide modern diagnostic, treatment, and rehabilitation facilities, hospitals may become so routine-oriented that individual patients and their need for nursing are submerged by routine practices. The task of each nurse in a hospital nursing situation is to make certain that each patient is provided with individualized nursing care and that the hospital system is adaptable to the nursing system for the individual patient. Routines are necessary, but they are not necessarily valid or justifiable if they interfere with the accomplishment of health goals and nursing goals for patients.

Other resident care facilities, such as extended care facilities and nursing homes, present some of the same advantages and disadvantages to nursing that the hospital presents. Routine service, large numbers of persons to be given care during the same time period, inadequate numbers of nurses, nurses with inadequate preparation, or the absence of nurses often militate against effective nursing in extended care facilities. Courtesy, kindness, and help from nurses in assuring patients that health care facilities and services are for their benefit are important in securing effective utilization of community facilities.

Other community facilities, such as clinics or day or night care health centers, serve patients who are at home for some part of the day. Nursing care of patients who come to these centers must take into consideration the possible need to adjust factors in the home environment to the patient's system of self-care or the need for the patient to make adjustments to the home situation. Hazards of travel, the time required for travel, available modes of travel, and costs require consideration.

Patients who are given nursing care in their own homes are in their accustomed environments. The environment is new for the nurse, however. A nurse who gives care to patients in their homes may be a staff member of an agency that provides home care nursing services. The agency may be a community health agency or a hospital that provides home care services. Such nurses have available to them equipment provided by the agency and may call upon the agency for other types of health care services needed by persons receiving nursing.

Persons who are in permanent or temporary residence in health care institutions such as hospitals, who may require nursing as well as other forms of health care, will require a range of services due purely to their status as residents. Figure 7-1 identifies services that health care institutions such as hospitals and nursing homes should provide for persons under health care, health care providers and other workers, and visitors.

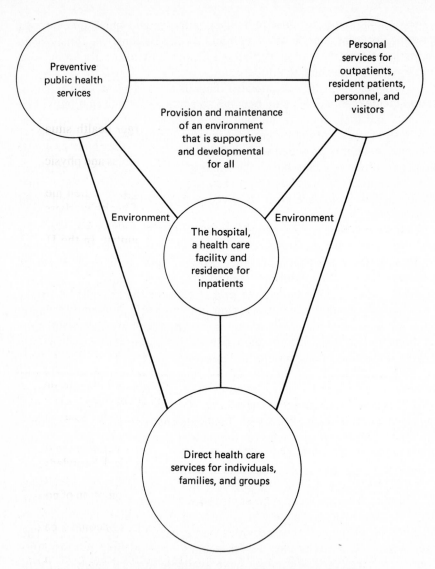

Figure 7-1 Service operations of hospitals and other health care facilities.

Whenever and wherever numbers of persons come or are brought together in common facilities (e.g., clinics), preventive public health services are essential for their protection. Ideally, an institution will maintain a supportive and developmental environment for all who come within its walls. The responsibility for the continued provision and maintenance of preventive public health services rests primarily with health care institution executives and administrators. All residence care and health care workers and other personnel, however, as well as patients and visitors, should participate in the fulfillment of this responsibility. Public health services are concerned with the protection of populations.

VARIATIONS IN MEDICAL CARE
AND OTHER FORMS OF HEALING

Variations in nursing situations that are parts of larger health situations arise from the number and kinds of health workers contributing care or service to patients. In some situations there are only nurses and physicians, but in others there are many types of health workers. For example, when persons suffer from an illness of undetermined origin or when medical treatment is complex, a large number and a variety of health workers may be involved. Forms of health care vary from one part of the world to another and, in some instances, within the same country. In the United States, the predominant form of health care is derived from scientific medicine as it has developed in the Western world.

This form of health care has traditionally had as its focus *disease*, which is defined as an abnormal biological process with characteristic symptoms. The modern concept of disease describes it as a process involving alterations in human structure or functioning including integrated human functioning. The modern concept of disease also includes the concept that a specific disease has more than a single cause (concept of multiple causation). Medical scientists identify, describe, and name unique diseases, that is, distinct pathological processes. Descriptions include the sequential series of changes that have been observed in individuals suffering from particular diseases.

The increasing knowledge about disease has been complemented by substantial increases of physiological and psychological knowledge of value to physicians and other health workers in the diagnosis, treatment, and prevention of disease and in the maintenance and promotion of normal development and functioning. Information about the prevention of disease and the maintenance and promotion of good health has become a part of the general culture. Thus health has come into focus in scientific medicine not just as something to be restored but as a desirable state to be maintained. As a result, the social and economic dimensions of health and health care have been given increased prominence.

At the present stage of its development, scientific medicine includes what has become known as *preventive medicine*, which is defined as "the science and art of preventing disease, prolonging life and promoting physical and mental health and efficiency . . . through intercepting disease processes by community and individual action."[7] Preventive medicine

[7]Hugh Rodman Leavell, E. Gurney Clark, et al., *Preventive Medicine for the Doctor in His Community*, McGraw-Hill, New York, 1965, p. 11.

recognizes (1) disease as a process of multiple causation, (2) the relationship of the process to disease agents, living or nonliving, (3) human characteristics, and (4) human responses to internal and external disease-producing stimuli.[8]

The physician is recognized as the practitioner of scientific medicine, whose functions in society include the diagnosis and treatment of disease and its effects. Medical diagnosis, the identification of natural causes and natural effects of disease, precedes treatment. Medical treatment is extended not only to the cure and control of disease processes and the restoration of health and alleviation of symptoms, but also to the prevention of disease and to overcoming defects and disability. Physicians in private or group practice of medicine perform these measures for individuals and families. Other physicians may be associated with various organizations, such as hospitals or business and industrial organizations, to supply care to the clients or the members of these organizations and sometimes to their families.

Medical care refers to the care given to individuals by physicians. The term is sometimes used in a broader sense for services to individuals by agencies and members of the various health professions and occupations—hospitals, physicians, dentists, nurses, and pharmacists. Nursing as a health care service is properly referred to as a part of medical care when the term *medical care* is used with this broader meaning.[9]

Nonmedical systems of health care exist in addition to the scientific system of medical care commonly practiced in the United States. Some systems have a basis other than disease. Christian Science healing is an example of a nonmedical system of health care. It is a religion with a basic tenet that when people are sick their thinking is at fault and that correct thinking will restore health.[10] This religious movement continues to satisfy the needs of some persons in their sufferings due to ill health.

Two other forms of healing practiced in the United States are chiropractic and naturopathy. Chiropractic is a system of health care based upon the belief that the central nervous system controls all the body systems and physiological functions and that malfunction of the nervous system will interfere with and impair the functions of the remaining body systems. Forms of treatment used by the chiropractor (doctor of chiropractic, D.C.) include vertebral manipulation and adjustment therapy to achieve normal nerve functioning, nutrition and dietary guidance, physical therapy, and counseling. Naturopathy is a form of healing practiced by the naturopath (doctor of naturopathy, N.D.). In the past, naturopaths

[8]Ibid., p. 15.
[9]Ibid., p. 12.
[10]Henry E. Sigerist, *Civilization and Disease,* University of Chicago Press, Phoenix Books, Chicago, 1943, p. 144.

depended upon water, air, sunlight, exercise, rest, diet, and moral standards in some prescribed combination for the treatment of individual cases of ill health, but they now include other forms of treatment, such as ultraviolet and x-ray therapy and colonic irrigations.

Primitive systems of medicine still exist in some areas of the world. Some of these systems are based on beliefs about mysterious or evil forces in nature that can cause illness. In cultures where beliefs in witchcraft, spirit possession, and evil forces in the natural environment exist, rules and rituals have been developed to protect people and their possessions from evil forces and to treat diseases. The medicine man and the witch doctor occupy important positions in primitive societies with duties that go beyond the diagnosis and cure of disease. Societies that are in a state of transition may have systems combining primitive medicine and scientific medicine. Medical doctors in some instances have learned to work effectively with practitioners of primitive medicine to improve the health of the people. Systems of primitive medicine contain some practices that are effective in the treatment of disease. In some systems of primitive medicine, religious, magical, and rational measures are combined.[11]

In the United States and other countries where scientific medicine is practiced, some individuals and groups practice *folk medicine* by using home remedies within the setting of the family or the neighborhood. These systems of folk medicine develop empirically from the observations and experiences of families and societies in the diagnosis and treatment of common illnesses and injuries. Beliefs are passed on from one generation to another.

Current practices of physicians and other health workers have come under attack within the framework of a general strain in the relations of "science and technology to society."[12] These attacks come both from within and outside the health care disciplines. Some are constructive and some are destructive. Turning away from science and technology has resulted in the increased popularity of astrology, magic, spiritism, adherence to various belief systems including the Eastern religions, and seeking non-Western forms of medical treatment (e.g., acupuncture).

Health Workers

Public Health Practitioners   Medical science and practice are focused on health maintenance and promotion as well as on disease. The medical doctor and the dentist are recognized in the United States as health practitioners concerned with the diagnosis and control of disease in individuals. With the growing emphasis on health, however, some medical doctors

[11]Ibid., pp. 131–132.
[12]Steven Louis Goldman, "Present Strains in the Relations between Science, Technology and Society," *Science, Technology, and Human Values,* vol. 4, Spring 1979, p. 4.

and dentists have channeled their efforts toward the promotion of health for groups and whole communities and specialize in preventive medicine and dentistry. Many kinds of trained health workers and lay persons as well engage in the maintenance and promotion of health on a community basis. These workers are often referred to as public health or community health workers. They have close ties to local governmental or nongovernmental groups organized for health promotion. At the state, city, and county levels qualified physicians fill the positions of health officer or health commissioner.

Persons with special education in the theory and practice of public health and preventive medicine come from a number of fields. Some physicians, dentists, and professional nurses specialize in the field of public health. Other specialists in public health include epidemiologists, health educators, nutritionists, food sanitarians, sanitary engineers, and statisticians (who work with morbidity and mortality information). All contribute professional effort toward the improvement of community health. Since health is so closely allied with the culture of the community, with physical, technological, and social conditions, and with personal and family living, community health workers should know the major facets of the environment and the community life.

The focus in professional community health work is the health of the community. This focus is in contrast to a focus on the health of a specific individual or family. Health workers concerned with the health of individuals and families may also be concerned with the health of the community, but their immediate focus is the individual or family rather than the community. The health workers who serve individuals and families by attending to their different needs for the prevention, diagnosis, treatment, and control of disease are described below.

Medical Doctors   Medical doctors are classified according to their specialties. Specialization is the limiting or concentration of effort toward accomplishing selected results using specific techniques. Some physicians engage in the general practice of medicine, rendering medical care to individuals and families with regard to the maintenance and promotion of health and the diagnosis and treatment of illnesses that do not demand modes of diagnosis or therapy for which specialized preparation is required. Specialization in medical practice has increased rapidly in the United States. Proportionately more graduates of medical schools have been choosing to limit their practice of medicine to special competencies in the diagnosis and treatment of particular health problems.[13]

[13]Iago Galdston, *Medicine in Transition*, University of Chicago Press, Chicago, 1965, pp. 113–114 and 159–160.

Approved specialty boards provide qualifying examinations for physicians who fulfill certain requirements and certify those who are successful. Certification helps to ensure the public that the physician specialist has proper capabilities. Areas of medical specialization include:

Anesthesiology
Dermatology
Internal medicine
Internal medicine subspecialties
   Allergy
   Cardiovascular disease
   Gastroenterology
   Pulmonary disease
Obstetrics and gynecology
Ophthalmology
Otolaryngology
Pathology
Pediatrics
Pediatric subspecialties
   Pediatric allergy
   Pediatric cardiology

Physical medicine and
   rehabilitation
Preventive medicine
Psychiatry and neurology
Radiology
Surgery
Colon and rectal surgery
Neurological surgery
Orthopedic surgery
Plastic surgery
Thoracic surgery
Urology

In the United States, medical doctors are licensed by the individual states in which they choose to practice. Boards of examiners prescribe the standards of education and qualification for the practice of medicine within the state. In addition, physicians are expected to conduct themselves according to the standards of professional medical practice set by the medical profession and the local medical society. When a physician becomes a member of the medical staff in a hospital, he or she also is responsible for adhering to and promoting high standards of medical practice and care established by that institution. Not all physicians, however, have a hospital association, which would permit them to care for their patients who require hospitalization. When patients of physicians without hospital privileges require hospitalization, it may be necessary for these physicians to refer their patients directly to a hospital or to a physician who is a member of a hospital medical staff.

During wars, disasters, and other emergencies, when qualified physicians may be scarce or unavailable, health workers trained in the use of selected medical care techniques may be called upon to perform some of the functions ordinarily performed by physicians. Medical corpsmen in the armed forces and civilian defense personnel are examples of these workers.

Dentists   Dentists (doctor of dental surgery, D.D.S., or doctor of dental medicine, D.D.M.) diagnose and treat diseases of the mouth, teeth, jaws, and gums and promote oral health. The dentist thus has an important role in comprehensive medical care for individuals and families. Some dentists engage in the general practice of dentistry. Others specialize, for example, the dental surgeon; the orthodontist, who is concerned with the prevention and correction of irregularities of the teeth; and the periodontist, who diagnoses and treats diseases of the gums and the structures that support the teeth. Dentists who specialize in the preventive aspects of dentistry in public health have important roles in community health programs.

Osteopaths   Doctors of osteopathy (D.O.) practice osteopathic medicine. Although this system of medicine emphasizes the importance of the musculoskeletal system in total body health, it includes the medical sciences and technologies that relate to the promotion of health and the prevention, diagnosis, and treatment of disease. Osteopaths, like medical doctors, must be licensed in the state where they practice. In some states, the graduates of medical colleges and osteopathic colleges take the same examination for state certification and licensure. In some communities, osteopaths maintain hospitals; in others, they use the same hospital facilities the medical doctors use.

Other Specialists   Doctors of podiatry (Pod. D.) or chiropody (D.S.C.) care for the feet in health and disease and detect conditions that should be referred to a medical doctor. Podiatry and chiropody are considered to be synonymous terms by the American Podiatry Association, the national organization of these specialists.

The optometrist (O.D.) identifies visual defects and prescribes corrective glasses or some forms of visual training.

Paramedical and Technical Service Personnel   The practice of scientific medicine requires a number of paramedical and technical services. Paramedical services contribute to some one aspect of medical practice. The major paramedical services are physical therapy, occupational therapy, speech therapy, and some of the services of medical social workers. The various paramedical services use specialized diagnostic and treatment techniques requiring skilled personnel.

Nutritionists and dietitians may have important roles in care directed toward the prevention, cure, or control of disease, working with both the physician and the patient whenever dietary treatment is involved. Clinical psychologists also perform functions that contribute to the diagnosis and treatment of mental and emotional disorders through psychological testing, counseling, and other therapeutic techniques.

In addition to the above services, other highly specialized technical services are essential in the physician's use of diagnostic and therapeutic measures. Physicians diagnosing and determining the course of a disease or a disorder and the effects of therapy require not only the efforts of physicians who are specialists in pathology but also the services of chemists, physicists, and clinical laboratory technicians. The physician in his or her medical practice may also require the services of other physicians who specialize in roentgenology (radiologists) and technicians skilled in the use of x-rays and other types of radiation.

HEALTH CARE SITUATIONS:
THE PATIENT'S POINT OF VIEW

Patients see their health care situations from their own unique perspectives. Their education, experience, feeling and attitudes about life and people, knowledge of health care and attitudes toward it color their views. Patients' insights about their own health care needs, the meaning they attach to presenting signs and symptoms, and their awareness of their ability or inability to engage in effective required self-care and to work cooperatively with nurses and physicians is essential information for nurses to have and use in helping patients. Individual nurses should develop approaches that are helpful to them in grasping quickly the views of individual patients about their health care situations and in identifying the interests and concerns of patients.

A woman being interviewed by a nurse-midwife about her obstetrical experiences[14] expressed the following views of herself in relation to her first pregnancy: (1) not having knowledge of what to do because of the pregnancy; (2) requiring time to formulate and express questions to ask the nurse and the obstetrician; (3) being able to cope with some but not all of the demands for self-care and self-management during the pregnancy; (4) being in need of learning to live as a woman who is pregnant and who is in labor, to relate to health care professionals, and to provide infant care; (5) being ready or not ready to learn at specific times. The woman noted that she was well educated, intelligent, and occupationally effective. She was aware of her own limitations for effective action within the health care situations associated with her first pregnancy. Time was viewed as a relevant factor.

The following account of a woman who underwent surgery to correct structural deformities of both feet provides an example of a period of

[14]Taken from the record of an interview conducted by Mary E. Fitzpatrick.

hospitalization and presents a patient's perspective of a surgical operation. It is important for nurses to understand that health-deviation self-care requisites are associated with the processes of preparation for surgery, the effects and results of the use of anesthesia, the tissues, organs, or organ system involved, the nature of the pathology, and the operative procedure and surgical techniques used.

Before Hospital Admission

My doctor sent me to see Dr. Robert Enders, head of the orthopedic section of a nearby clinic, because I had a severe pain in my right shoulder. After he examined my shoulder, Dr. Enders said that I had an acute attack of bursitis but that no treatment other than rest and some slight medication for the pain should be used. He had x-rays taken and said that there were no deposits of calcium.

I told Dr. Enders that I had been having a similar pain in the second toe of my left foot and asked if I also had bursitis in that region. I told him that in addition to the acute pain in the second toe, both feet were painful. Dr. Enders asked to see my feet. When he saw them, he said that x-rays should be taken. He told me after this first examination that the pain I had in my left foot was due to a distorted toe caused by a bunion in the joint of the big toe.

When he asked me how long I had been troubled with bunions, I explained that about four years earlier I had started to wear a pair of shoes prescribed for metatarsal support. After wearing the shoes for several hours I removed them because of pain. I noted upon removing the shoes that I had suffered a hemorrhage of both big toes, probably due to unusual pressure on the joints. I did not wear the shoes again. The joints continued to bother me, and it was obvious that my feet were gradually becoming worse—more crippled and more painful.

After the x-rays were taken and a more detailed examination made, Dr. Enders advised surgery to correct the crippled condition of my feet and relieve the pain. At this time I was able to maintain my normal schedule, but I wondered how long I could continue to do so. I was quite willing to undergo the surgery Dr. Enders advised.

Preoperative Days

I was admitted to the hospital on May 13. Upon arrival at my room I met a very friendly, motherly looking woman who was the secretary of the floor. The room was a pleasant one with west and south exposures. It was immaculate and well furnished and uncluttered.

I was in my room just a few seconds when a nurse came in and fastened a bracelet around my left wrist. It was an identification bracelet of clear, white plastic on which were typed my name and my number.

After I had been in bed about five minutes a number of doctors began examining me. Although I was there only for foot surgery, I was given a complete physical examination. I had many tests—blood, urinalysis, heart, reflexes, and lung.

Shortly after the first doctor left me, the secretary of the floor came into the room, cut off the white wristlet, and put on a coral-colored one. When I asked her why she was changing the wristlet, she said that all allergic persons wore coral-colored wristlets and that a nurse would not give medication to a patient wearing a coral bracelet without checking the card [medication card] against the medical order.

When I looked at the inside of my bracelet I found the words "morphine," and "codeine." These were the two drugs that I had told the doctor I could not tolerate as they made me feel nauseous.

I was not to undergo surgery until Friday and did not expect that I would see anyone from the operating room before Thursday. I was mistaken. About 5 o'clock of that first day, two nursing students came to prepare my feet and legs. They were quite efficient about their work, very friendly and cheerful, and won me at once by their enthusiasm for nursing. They obviously were accustomed to working together. They did their work thoroughly and, I thought, with almost no wasted motion.

I discovered that preparing a person for an operation like this involved soaping and shaving my legs from the toes to the middle of the thighs. I asked why they had to shave such a large area when the operation was going to be on my feet. They smiled and said that it was very important to be sure that more than the actual operative area be surgically clean. One explained that the procedure would be performed again the following day by a nurse and immediately prior to surgery in the operating room by my surgeon.

My one big concern at this time was whether I would be confined to my bed after the first preparation when the surgery was still thirty-six hours away. The nursing students said that I would be able to bathe and live "normally" until the second preparation, which would take place the next evening. With that, they cleaned and packed their equipment, said goodbye, and left.

My dinner was brought in and I ate everything. Later, a young aide came to pick up my tray. I talked to her for a while. I had many conversations with this young girl during my hospital stay.

After 7 o'clock, a doctor from the anesthesia department came to explain the procedure. I immediately asked what anesthetic would be used for the operation. The anesthetist said that I would be given sodium pentothal for the anesthetic and probably would be given Demerol for pain, since he had noted from my chart that I was allergic to codeine and morphine. I thanked him and told him I had no more questions.

The head nurse visited with me. I asked about the Catholic chaplain and she explained the arrangements for visits from him. After the head nurse left, I took a bath and returned to my room. After I got back into bed, the nurse assigned to me asked about my needs. Later the head nurse came in to see if I needed anything. I said I didn't need a thing, and around 9:30 I went to sleep.

I awakened at 6:15 A.M. I got up and went to the bathroom. When I returned, the night nurse came in for a last check before going off duty. She said she had been in several times during the night and that I had been asleep each time.

At 7:30 a nurse took my temperature and then got out the water basins to get me ready for breakfast. I washed my face and brushed my teeth. After finishing, I settled back to wait for breakfast. The doctor had not yet put me on a planned 1200-calorie diet, so I had a good breakfast—fruit, hot cereal, bacon, scrambled eggs, a piece of toast, and two cups of coffee.

After breakfast the nurse came back to ask me if I wanted to have a bath. I told her that since I was still able to walk around, I would go down the hall and have a tub bath. While I was gone, my bed was remade and the room straightened up.

At noon my 1200-calorie diet began, and the tray did not look half as plentiful for lunch as it had for breakfast. The food, however, was very good. I had clear soup, salad without dressing, a half slice of bread, a slice of roast beef, a small glass of milk, and a cup of tea. After lunch the nurse asked me if I wanted to have a back rub before taking a nap. I said I would. We soon began talking about a concert that was to be given the following week. Later that afternoon my sister Mary and a friend of hers came to visit. Mary told me that she would be in again before surgery on Friday morning.

Thursday evening after supper, two different nursing students came from the operating room. They performed the skin preparation all over again, scrubbing, shaving, and cleansing the whole area with alcohol. They asked me not to get out of bed again.

The head nurse came in shortly after they left and asked me if I had any questions or apprehensions about the surgery. She said she would talk to me about them if I had. I told her that the doctor had explained the operation to me. She then suggested that I try to settle down for the night early, as it was important to have a good night's sleep before surgery. She came back a little later, after I had washed, and gave me a good back rub and a sleeping pill, and I settled for the night. During the night, I woke up a couple of times. Since I had been asked not to get out of bed, instead of going to the bathroom I rang for the nurse. That night I met the head night nurse who was very helpful and kind during my stay.

Day of Surgery

The next morning I awoke early to find the nurse at my bedside, ready to give me some "pre-op" medication. She was a bit concerned about whether I would be able to take medicine when she knew I wanted to receive communion. I assured her it was all right. I then waited for Father Bailey. Fifteen minutes after Father Bailey left she returned with more medication and advised me to lie as still as possible. Just as I was becoming extremely groggy, my sister Mary came in for a visit.

Almost immediately the head nurse came in with an orderly, I believe. They moved me from my bed to the cart and wheeled me down the hall. By this time I was too far gone to know exactly when we got into the elevator to go down to the operating room floor or when we got off. I remember talking with Dr. Enders. Shortly afterward I felt a sharp jab in my left arm; that was the last I knew.

When I came to, I was back in my own bed, violently ill. Someone was supporting my forehead and holding a basin close to me. I couldn't understand why I was so sick because I hadn't eaten any food. It was all dry retching. I had a tremendous urge to vomit; but when I did, nothing came up. After three or four attempts at this, I fell back on my pillow, completely exhausted and soaking wet. The nurse mopped my brow and face and changed my gown. This went on all day. In between, I had moments of oblivion still due, I suppose, to the anesthetic. While the pain in my feet was very bad, I was so conscious of the feeling of nausea and the urgency to vomit that I forgot the pain.

After what seemed like several hours, I remember the nurse sponging me and rubbing my back. This brought me some relief, and I dozed for a few minutes. During the day the doctor had been in to see what he could do about curtailing the nausea. Since they had not given me any of the narcotics to which I was allergic, he could not understand why I was having so much nausea. He ordered injections of a medication that was supposed to stop vomiting. I also remember that Mary visited me. The retching and heaving continued until that night. At one point, I vomited a great deal of bile. That brought some relief. I didn't realize that the gastrointestinal tract would secrete juices even when I had not eaten any food.

When I came to after the operation, I was very conscious of acute discomfort in my right elbow and shoulder. I could see below the short sleeve of the hospital gown the vivid color of the solution used to paint an operative area. I asked about it, and the nurse told me that the doctor had injected both the elbow and the shoulder while I was under the general anesthetic for the foot surgery in an attempt to ease the bursitis pain in the elbow and shoulder joints.

While I had discussed the problem with the doctor, I had not realized that he would be able to take care of the different areas at the same time. The discomfort of the injections wore off quickly, whereas the foot pain was intense for many days.

Postoperative Days

The nausea continued in varying degrees until about 6 o'clock in the morning when the nurse helped me to rinse my mouth. The nausea did not return for about two hours. About 8 o'clock that morning Dr. Enders came to see if there was any hope that the nausea would stop and to see how the pain in my feet was. Although the pain was severe, I was so exhausted by the nausea that I did not say much to him about the pain in my feet.

The day wore on. A nurse came in about 9:30 to bathe me, make my bed, and change my gown. She also took my temperature, gave me a back rub, and left.

About 11 o'clock the nurse returned to see if I could tolerate a little weak tea. I thought I would try it. I did and managed to keep it down. We felt that the nausea was pretty much at an end. The head nurse came in every two or three hours to see whether I needed medication for the pain in my feet. As I was somewhat concerned about the possibility of prolonging the nausea, I refrained from taking medication very often. As a result, the pain built up to a frightening degree. Saturday afternoon passed in this way, with concerned care from the nurses. The pain was severe. At supper time I had a cup of weak tea, which was all I could try.

The nurses gave me Demerol for the pain, which was like water so far as I was concerned. I felt absolutely no change in the intensity of the pain. One of Dr. Enders' assistants and my medical doctor came to see me. A new medication in the form of pills was ordered for pain this time. They brought relief, but only for about thirty minutes.

Later, Dr. Enders came in. He cut open the bandages and splints and discovered that my feet were swollen beyond his expectation for surgery of this kind. He said that much pain could have been eliminated had the bandages not become so tight from the swelling. After my feet had recovered a little bit from the pressure, he put new bandages on them again. During that time I was flat on the bed, with my feet on a pillow. I had a cradle over them for the first few days. Later the doctor removed the cradle, and the nurses put a board at the foot of the bed to keep covers off my feet.

Monday morning the aides from the x-ray department took me down to be x-rayed. They had me slip over from my bed onto the cart. Then they rolled me down to the department for pictures of my feet. When I returned I was wringing wet and utterly exhausted, even though I had not exerted myself other than to slip onto and off the cart.

Later Dr. Enders told me that the x-rays were good. He thought that I would be able to get out of bed and sit in the chair. He wanted me to do this without putting any pressure on the front parts of my feet. When the nurses came in, we managed to do this first by having me sit on the side of the bed. I dangled my legs for a few minutes. Then two of the nurses lifted me down to the floor with the heels of my feet touching. They backed me into a chair. They apparently were used to this kind of operation because moving me from the bed to the chair presented no great problem to them.

From this point on I felt that my recovery started. I continued to have pain, sometimes severe pain, but it never again approached the pain of the first days. Every four hours they gave me pills, and while I felt relief for only a very short time, the pills enabled me to get through the day without too much discomfort. That evening I enjoyed my meal for the first time and was able to eat a large portion of my dinner.

After dinner the nurse came in and saw to my comfort for the evening. I spent that evening, as I was to spend many other evenings, lying in relative comfort, looking at the sunset. I couldn't read. Friends came and I enjoyed their visits.

The days took on a pattern. The nurse took my temperature. The aide brought me two pans so that I could wash and also brush my teeth before breakfast. Then an aide came in with fresh water, took out the pans, and straightened the room. By the time the breakfast trays were ready, I was refreshed and my room was in order.

After breakfast one of the nurses came in to see if I was ready to start my bath. They helped me each day with my back and legs. Two of them got me up. They never let me get up without helping me. Each day I was able to do a little more about helping myself get up and get down. While sitting up, I always had my feet on a footstool that had a pillow on it to make my feet a little higher than the chair. The aide made the bed and straightened up the room. Usually while I was in the chair, the maid came in and cleaned the room. The doctors visited in the morning, questioned me, and examined my feet. The chaplain came each day.

The second day I was up, the doctor sent the physiotherapist to measure me for crutches and to teach me how to walk with them. I found it very difficult to balance myself on my heels with the crutches. The physiotherapist and the doctor decided that if I could learn to walk with a "skiing motion," without putting any pressure on the front of my feet, I would not have to use the crutches. This I learned to do very quickly with the physiotherapist's help by holding onto the furniture as I went around the room.

I walked each morning. For the first three or four days the nurses would not let me walk without having someone with me. I went out in the hall each day to walk because I couldn't get any practice in my room, which had little walking area. Once each morning and once each afternoon I would walk the length of about four rooms. When Mary or my friends came in the afternoon, one of them would accompany me; and in the morning one of the nurses would take me for a walk. I didn't walk out in the hall alone until the day I left the hospital.

While walking, I had to give all my attention to keeping my toes up. It was such an unnatural walk. I felt pain all the way up the front of my legs from holding my toes this way.

By this time I was enjoying my food and wishing I had more of it. I ate everything they gave me. I was on the 1200-calorie diet because both the doctor and I thought it would be wise for me to lose some weight while I was in the hospital. A weight loss, which I could well afford, would result in a lighter burden for my feet.

I did not sleep well all the time I was in the hospital because I was so tense. I think the tenseness was due to the pain. The pain was constant, but not like the terrible pain of the first few days. In fact, I found my days quite pleasant. The surroundings were peaceful and pleasant. Most important, I had wonderful care. No matter how busy the doctors or nurses were or how involved anything was, I received sympathetic attention. You do not get this in many hospitals from what I have heard from others and have experienced myself.

The patients on my end of the floor were friendly. I would speak to them in the hall, and some came into my room to visit. One lady would come in and sit with me sometimes for thirty minutes. There was another lady who had been having all sorts of difficult tests and who was going to have chest surgery. She came to see me two or three times.

One evening the ambulatory patients asked the nurse on the floor if they could use the room across from mine to play cards. They played canasta until about 9:30 and had a marvelous time. When the nurse came to talk with me that night she told me she had come down two or three times to ask them to be quieter because some patients had just been returned from surgery. She said that she regretted having to do it because she felt it was very important for the patients to have recreation.

The day before I went home, Dr. Enders came in with his assistant and a nurse to remove the bandages and stitches. He took the stitches out of my left foot, and his first assistant took the stitches out of my right foot at the same time. During their work they discussed another patient's surgical procedure, I guess to divert my attention. They didn't succeed. Afterwards, they sponged my feet with "orange" liquid and put on new splints and fresh bandages. Doctor Enders told me to report to the clinic in two weeks for x-rays and new bandages and said I could go home the next day.

Commentary

The foregoing excerpts from a patient's story reveal a person who was observant of details, who was interested in people and what they did and said, and who had experienced both hospitalization and surgery on a previous occasion. Because of this previous experience it was evident that the patient had certain expectations about what would occur and what various persons would do and when they would do it. However, the new experience was not entirely in accord with her past experience. A patient who had not had surgery would not have expectations based on a past life experience; lack of knowledge or awareness of the unpleasant experience of another person might result in anxiety and apprehension. A previous surgical experience of an extremely unpleasant nature might cause the same effect.

The health care situation presented according to the patient's point of view is analyzed to bring out important positions and roles. No comment will be made about the quality of the services that were performed to meet the health care requirements of the person telling the story. This is a patient's account and is accepted as such.

AN ANALYSIS OF THE PATIENT'S HEALTH CARE SITUATION

Medical Care

In the patient's story just narrated, four medical doctors are mentioned: the surgeon, the surgeon's assistant, the patient's medical doctor (who was a specialist in internal medicine), and the anesthetist. There were other behind-the-scenes specialists whom the patient did not mention—a radiologist, for example, who reported the evidence about the condition of the bones of the patient's feet as revealed in the x-rays. If tissue were removed from the patient during surgery, it probably was examined by a pathologist. Pathologists and radiologists have very specialized roles in the diagnosis and treatment of disease. What these specialists do facilitates the work of the physician.

In her story the patient mentioned the aides from the x-ray department who were responsible for transporting her to and from this department. There were also the x-ray technicians who positioned her and took the x-ray pictures. Someone had to develop the x-ray film after the pictures were taken. In addition, clinical laboratory technicians took samples of blood from the patient and performed various blood tests and urinalysis. Again, reports of the findings were prepared and transmitted for entry in the patient's record.

In this health care situation the orthopedic surgeon had the central role since the form of medical treatment was corrective surgery on the patient's deformed feet. He could not have performed effectively without the help of his surgical assistant, the anesthetist, the radiologist, and the operating room staff. The patient's relationship with her medical doctor was of longer duration, however; he saw the patient during her period of hospitalization but was not responsible for the diagnosis, treatment, or rehabilitation measures related to the pathological condition of her feet. When a patient has more than one doctor, it is important for his or her welfare that the doctors in attendance coordinate their efforts. The patient's story contains evidence to indicate that she had confidence and trust in the doctors who gave her care and that she accepted them without fear or apprehension. The patient's story does not include the events just before, during, and immediately after surgery since she was anesthetized and unaware. The following paragraph describes those events in general terms.

In the modern hospital, surgical procedures are performed in specialized facilities referred to as the operating room, the surgical suite, or the surgical theater. The surgeon works under controlled conditions that maintain a state of maximum surgical asepsis in the operating area, thereby minimizing the possibility of wound infections. The prevention of infection is an essential aspect of surgical treatment since nearly all surgical techniques involve the use of instruments to penetrate body cavities and often require the incising and suturing of tissue. Precautions are also taken to prevent explosions or fires when explosive or flammable gases or other unstable materials are used in operating rooms.

In planning for and in performing surgery, each person involved bears responsibility for his or her particular part in the surgical procedure. The surgeon and one or more assistants, an anesthetist, surgical nurses, operating room technicians, the pathologist, the roentgenologist, x-ray and laboratory technicians, and other types of specialized workers may be involved. Nurses who are responsible for the care of a patient prior to surgery have an important role in helping the patient become "ready" for surgery. According to the patient's story, x-ray personnel and clinical laboratory technicians had direct contact with her. In some medical care situations, pathologists and radiologists may also have direct contact with the patient and with her physician, but there is no evidence of this in the patient's story.

It is the physician's responsibility to write medical orders for the specific clinical laboratory tests and x-ray examinations he or she deems necessary in the medical diagnosis and care of the patient. These orders become a part of the patient's medical record. These tests and examinations are also necessary so that the physician may follow the course of a disease process or evaluate the results of specific types of therapy or treatment. In the patient's story the x-ray examinations following the operation were of the evaluation type. This patient also had a diagnostic series of x-ray examinations of her feet prior to the decision that corrective surgery was the treatment of choice.

The orders a physician writes for tests and examinations must be transmitted to the appropriate department of the hospital or, if the patient is not hospitalized, to the public or private clinic or laboratory where the tests or examinations will be done. When the orders are received by the appropriate department, they become indicators of the work that must be done by the personnel of that department. Transmitting such orders to and within departments involves activities of a communicative and clerical type—work that can be done effectively by responsible, trained secretaries or clerks. In some institutions, these duties are considered the proper work of nurses. Although this work has and continues to be done by nurses, it is in no sense nursing. It is clerical administrative work related solely to the transmitting of medical orders to coordinate the work of the physician with the work of persons who aid physicians in their care of patients. Nursing does have a role in preparing patients for tests and examinations, but this role relates to assisting the patient to perform needed preparatory measures such as taking prescribed medications, the cleansing of the lower intestinal tract, the withholding of food, or eating a special type of food prior to a test or examination.

In the patient's story, both the hospital dietitian and the physiotherapist had roles in the prescribed care of the patient. There was a problem of excessive weight, which was controlled through a 1200-calorie diet. The dietician's role was to assure the patient a nutritious diet, selected in light of the limited calories and the type of surgical procedure performed. The role of the physiotherapist was to assist the patient in walking under unnatural conditions, in this case, without disturbing the structures of the foot on which surgical reconstruction had been done. The physiotherapist was also responsible for assisting in the prevention of further defect and disability as the result of an unnatural manner of walking. In her story, the patient indicated knowledge of the reasons for the low-calorie diet and the manner of walking she was directed to use.

Nursing Care

In the patient's story "nurses" and "head nurses" are mentioned as being there to assist her 24 hours of the day. The story indicates that the "head nurses" made evaluations and decisions and initiated or performed activities related to the nursing care of the patient that differed from those of other "nurses." One can conclude that both "head nurses" and "nurses" had responsibilities for care of the same patient. An aide was described as performing tasks such as the removal of trays on which meals were served and bringing and removing equipment and materials used in daily hygienic care. Nursing students from the operating room cleansed the skin of the patient's legs and feet preoperatively and gave directives about walking following each preparation. Other nursing students explained the surgical routine for skin preparation and responded to the patient's question about the reason for preparing such an extensive area.

From the viewpoint of the reason for the patient's hospitalization, the patient's experiences were divided into the preoperative period, the period of surgery, and the postoperative period. Prior to surgery and until the last surgical preparation, the patient attended to her own personal care needs. Meals were brought to her, and the other resources she needed were available to her as well. It should be noted that the patient followed the directive that she not get out of bed after the last cleansing of the skin of her legs and feet prior to surgery. The patient, although able to walk, followed the instruction to remain in bed, thus exercising voluntary restraint. She thereby indicated that she not only understood and accepted the directive but that she remembered it.

The head nurses and other nurses made themselves available to the patient during the preoperative period, although the patient was quite self-sufficient. We can therefore infer that they were indicating to her that she was not alone, that they were there to help her (supportive actions). At the same time they provided her with opportunities to ask questions or to express her apprehensions about the surgery. The evening before surgery the head nurse opened this matter by asking the patient if she felt any apprehensions concerning the surgical procedure. Then she proceeded to help the patient prepare for sleep.

The preanesthesia medications were given by the nurse on the morning of the surgery, initiating for the patient a period of limited awareness in which she was responsive to some but not all stimuli. In the operating room, a period of unconsciousness began and extended to the postoperative period when the patient became aware that she was in her hospital room and that "someone" was assisting her because of the postanesthesia nausea and vomiting. Periods of limited awareness and periods of oblivion continued for some time. During limited awareness, the patient was helpless, unable to act for herself or to protect herself from harm, though she apparently responded to the presence of persons who were with her. Again we may infer that the presence of the day head nurse, the patient's sister, her surgeon before surgery, and the "someone" who was with her following surgery was supportive and helped relieve the apprehension or fear that arises when one is alone and helpless.

During the postoperative period the patient had greater limitations with respect to self-care than she had before surgery. She also had new self-care needs as direct or indirect results of the surgery. The postoperative nausea, pain, and fatigue the patient described (1) demanded the attention of the nurses and the doctors, (2) necessitated the use of regulatory measures, some of which were medically prescribed, and (3) temporarily interfered with the normal intake of fluid and food and with the patient's accustomed activities such as reading and socializing.

Following surgery the patient was not able to walk naturally because her surgeon had directed her to put weight only on her heels. She required assistance in getting in and out of bed in following this directive. The patient also described the physical support, psychological support, and guidance extended by the nurses as they assisted her. In order to walk, the patient had to develop a new skill. Because she could not learn to use crutches following the directive of keeping weight off the "front parts" of her feet, she also had to learn a form of walking she referred to as the "skiing motion." The patient's story also indicates that the nurses were attentive to her as she "walked" and did not permit her to be alone. We can infer that they were concerned with preventing falls and with helping to increase her self-confidence through their presence.

The patient's story clearly points up her awareness that nurses were available to help her with the continuing aspects of her therapeutic care. The doctors visited, examined, prescribed, consulted with the patient and with other health workers, and performed specific measures (the surgery, the removal of the sutures). The physiotherapist assisted the patient with learning the new ambulatory skill. The x-ray technicians and laboratory technicians had contact with the patient because they had been directed to perform particular examinations and tests. The x-ray aides provided transportation service. The chaplain saw the patient daily. Her sister and friends visited her but it was the staff nurses and the head nurses who were present on a continuing basis. The story makes no mention of staff nurses and head nurses communicating with others who gave care to the patient, but there is evidence of cooperation and coordination among the nurses and among nurses and other health service workers who assisted the patient.

Health Care Requirements

In the patient's story a period of hospitalization for surgery is described in some detail. The patient who tells the story had experienced increasing difficulty with walking and standing because of a disabling condition of her feet. Through medical care prior to her hospitalization, the nature and extent of the structural and functional abnormalities of her feet were determined (the diagnosis), and this was followed by the physician's judgment that surgical treatment would be effective in overcoming the patient's disability. The surgeon advised the patient to undergo surgery, and she agreed. She was not informed that the bursitis of the shoulder and elbow joints would be treated at the same time.

The patient came to the hospital so that her surgeon could use the surgical facilities and equipment of the hospital and the benefits of the paramedical services, specialized diagnostic and therapeutic services, and nursing services that were necessary to her medical care. The treatment was surgical and required a general anesthetic, incision of the skin and subcutaneous tissues, orthopedic correction of the structural defects, closing and suturing the incised tissues, and bandaging and splinting of the feet. The continuing self-care that the patient had to exercise to help bring about the results desired from the surgery was control of weight distribution on her feet when she stood or walked. She needed both preparation (by the surgeon and the physiotherapist) and continuing assistance (by nurses) so that she could execute her role effectively. The control of weight distribution on her feet was an integral part of the postoperative treatment. Positioning of the lower extremities, splinting of the feet, and care of the surgical wounds were also integral parts of the postoperative therapy. The patient mentioned that she was also under dietary treatment to bring about a loss of weight that would benefit her general health and lessen the weight her feet would bear. The patient and the dietitian had roles in carrying out this therapy.

In her story the patient describes the swelling of the tissues of her feet following surgery—a clinical condition that the surgeon observed upon removal of the bandages. The pain and nausea the patient experienced were subjective; the retching and vomiting were observable by nurses and doctors. Tenseness, fatigue, and weakness were subjective experiences. The patient also experienced excessive perspiration in the early part of the postoperative period and after the effort necessary to get on and off the cart used by the x-ray personnel. Care measures were required because of all these occurrences, which were directly or indirectly related to the surgery.

Throughout, the doctors and nurses provided assistance and instituted health care measures to prevent accidental injuries and to prevent further defect and disability. Some preventive measures were control measures instituted for all hospital patients. For example, the identification wristlet of a special color was inscribed with the patient's name as a means of alerting personnel to her allergies and ensuring that she would not be given harmful drugs. The use of the cradle and the footboard following surgery was preventive, as was the assistance from nurses when the patient got in and out of bed and walked. The final preoperative medical examination and laboratory tests were done after she had been admitted to the hospital to determine her physical and psychological ability to undergo surgery. The conversation of the head nurse with the patient on the evening before surgery, her assistance in preparing for sleep on this same night, the availability of the nurses during the preoperative period, and the presence of the head nurse at the time the patient was being moved to surgery were in part preventive measures although they served other purposes.

It was evident in the patient's story that meeting her health care requirements took a large part of her day. Except for a few nights and days postoperatively, the daily life of the patient took on a regular pattern of daytime and evening activities and a period of sleep during the night hours. The patient lived through her period of hospitalization cooperatively by interacting with and coordinating her activities with doctors, nurses, and others who gave health and health-related care, with the chaplain, and with her relatives and friends. Experiencing new social relationships was a part of the hospital experience. Various aides, housekeeping maids, the ward secretary, and other hospitalized persons were also in contact with the patient.

The patient's hospital experiences were in part solitary and in part social. Regardless of the kindness and consideration shown to her by others and the actual care she received, it is evident that the patient lived through this experience as each person must live his or her life, unique and alone, while at the same time a member of a family or a community. During the relatively short duration of her hospitalization, the patient was a hospital resident with the position and role of patient within a complex health care system.

COOPERATION AND COORDINATION IN HEALTH CARE SITUATIONS

The achievement of health results for individuals is based in large part upon the capabilities and motivation of health service personnel and their willingness and ability to cooperate and to coordinate their efforts. To *cooperate* is to act jointly in achieving some common goal. A situation that requires cooperation or joint action of a number of persons sets up a demand that the persons acting together to reach a common goal regulate and combine their efforts so that action will be harmonious and will contribute to the achievement of the goal. This regulation and combination of effort is *coordination*.

If several people attempt to work toward a common goal but do so without coordination, duplication of effort, inefficiency, and even failure to achieve the goal may occur. Effective coordination of effort requires that persons involved reach a common understanding of their goal, know their respective roles in its achievement, perform in an agreed manner so that the activities will be properly related to the goal, and communicate developments and changes resulting from their actions whenever such information is necessary for the performance of other roles.

Learning to nurse includes learning to work in cooperation with patients and their families, other nurses, physicians, and other health care specialists. Nursing students and young nurses should have planned experiences designed to aid them in initiating and responding to contacts with other health workers as well as patients and their families. The language of the health and medical sciences facilitates communication between nurses and other health workers. Terms that are specific to a particular health service may need definition and explanation when used in interdisciplinary communication. The language of nursing is relatively undeveloped.

Beliefs of nurses and other health workers about their roles and the roles of others affect their interests and their willingness to function in cooperative relationships in health care situations. Some health workers have little insight about the specific characteristics of nursing and its significance in achieving health results. Nurses, on the other hand, because of their continuous relationship with a patient, often have considerable knowledge of the roles and contributions of other health workers. Nurses should have skill in representing to physicians, social workers, and others the characteristics of nursing and the nature of the health care contribution it can make in various types of health care situations.

The Health Team

Members of the various health or health-related services who give help to the same person are sometimes collectively referred to as a health team. A health team is an organized group of health workers who have roles related to meeting the health care needs of a patient or a group of patients. A team does not exist unless there are common goals, cooperative relationships, and coordinated activities. In many health care situations there are no health teams in the usual sense. Frequently, patients are cared for by a number of health workers who cooperate on a one-to-one basis with the patient and with other health workers. An organized health team enables its individual members to see their respective roles in relation to achievement of health results for a patient, to establish a group identity, and to afford authority to and to respect group members in relation to their roles and capabilities.

The formal establishment of a health team may be the only way or the preferred way for giving care or designing and managing care. Team functioning requires time and specialized effort on the part of each person involved. When health teams are not formally organized, cooperation and coordination of effort must be initiated by individual health workers.

Health teams are essential to performing some complex diagnostic and treatment measures. Often some members of these teams work with extremely complex machines or equipment that must be brought into a functional relationship with a patient (e.g., the heart-lung machine during open-heart surgery). Whenever team members work in face-to-face relationships or when linked by highly effective communication devices, coordination of effort is facilitated. Analysis of the roles, the relationships, and the specific activities of members of a health team (e.g., a surgical team preparing for and performing a surgical procedure for a patient in an operating room) is a helpful exercise toward understanding health team functioning.

SELECTED READINGS

Brownlee, Ann Templeton: *Community, Culture, and Care: A Cross-Cultural Guide for Health Workers,* C. V. Mosby, St. Louis, 1978.

Chavigny, Katherine Hill: "Microbial Infections in Hospitals: A Review of the Literature and Suggestions for Nursing Research," *International Journal of Nursing Studies,* vol. 14, 1977, pp. 37–47.

Chester, Thomas, et al.: "House-to-House, Community-Wide Chemoprophylaxis for Meningococcal Disease: An Aggressive Approach to Prevention," *American Journal of Public Health,* vol. 67, November 1977, pp. 1058–1062.

Clement, Jeanne A.: "The Helping Relationship: Choices and Dilemmas," *Issues in Mental Health Nursing,* vol. 1, Winter 1978, pp. 18–23.

Dunning, James, and Nora Dunning: "An International Look at School-Based Children's Dental Services," *American Journal of Public Health,* vol. 68, July 1978, pp. 664–668.

Gershenson, Charles P.: "Child Maltreatment, Family Stress, and Ecological Insult," *American Journal of Public Health,* vol. 67, July 1977, pp. 602–604.

Hilbert, Morton S.: "Prevention, Presidential Address," *American Journal of Public Health,* vol. 67, April 1977, pp. 353–356.

Horn, Barbara J., and Mary Ann Swain: *Development of Criterion Measures of Nursing Care, vols. 1 and 2,* University of Michigan and National Center for Health Services Research, U.S. Department of Commerce, National Technical Information Service, Springfield, Va., 1978, Publication 267-004 and 267-005.

Linn, Margaret W., et al.: "Patient Outcomes as a Measure of the Quality of Nursing Home Care," *American Journal of Public Health,* vol. 67, April 1977, pp. 334–337.

McGilloway, F. A., and Rev. Liam Donnally: "Religion and Patient Care: The Functionalist Approach," *Journal of Advanced Nursing,* vol. 2, January 1977, pp. 3–13.

Sinborg, Donald W., Barbara H. Starfield, and Susan D. Horn: "Physician and Non-physician Health Practitioners: The Characteristics of Their Practice and Their Relationships," *American Journal of Public Health,* vol. 68, January 1978, pp. 44–48.

Sowell, Thomas: "Ethnicity in a Changing America," *Daedalus,* vol. 107, Winter 1978, pp. 213–237.

Chapter 8

The Practice of Nursing

The art of nursing is expressed by individual nurses through their creativity in designing and providing nursing that is effective and satisfying for men, women, and children. It is grounded in knowledge and understanding of the characteristics of nursing as a personalized health service. Its practice requires knowledge about and understanding of the persons to be helped and served through nursing. The unit of a nurse's service may be an individual or a multiperson unit, but nursing ultimately is for human beings individually considered. Only individuals have self-care requisites to be met and the capabilities for meeting them.

DESCRIPTION AND REGULATION OF PRACTICE
Dimensions of Practice

The practice of nursing within social groups may be described along at least eight dimensions.

    1 The number of persons to be provided with nursing in relation to the prevalence of nursing requirements in a population and the incidence of occurrence of new nursing cases

194

2 The types of nursing systems that will be designed, produced, and managed for individuals or groups
3 The time when and the duration of time over which nursing will be provided
4 The place(s) where nursing will be provided
5 The means to be used in effecting nurse-patient contacts initially and throughout the period when nursing is required
6 Required contacts of nurses with and reasons for relationships with nurse colleagues, nurse assistants, nurse consultants and supervisors, and other health professionals
7 Materials and resources required for the production of nursing care and the means for their procurement, storage, preparation for use, and disposal or care after use
8 Means of payment for nursing

Nurses who engage in nursing practice must describe and regulate their practice along these eight dimensions. Nursing practice is work; sometimes it is laborious. Regulation of nursing practice is necessary for the well-being of nurses and of their patients.

Nurses have been and continue to be viewed as being without limits with respect to the numbers of persons they can care for and relate to and the kinds of nursing problems they can resolve. The limitations on what nurses can do, established by the kind of preparation for nursing they received, and their experiences have been largely ignored in practice settings. Also largely ignored are the needs of young nurses for career advancement and for working with nurses with advanced professional skill. Such views and practices are reflected in the standards of accrediting bodies that survey and accredit health care institutions and in the operational policies and practices of hospitals and other institutions where nurses provide care.

Some nurses have a tendency to associate their practice of nursing with the places where they provide nursing and with employing institutions if they are not self-employed. The focus on place and the focus on organizational membership, at times, supersede the focus on nursing. It is important for nurses who are employed in institutions to differentiate their nurse role from their employee role. Nurses, physicians, and other professionals contribute to the achievement of the purposes of health service institutions to the degree that they can and do provide health care, as defined by their respective domains, to case loads of patients. A person's ability to provide nursing and his or her status as nurse in a social group is not derived from the employing institution. The ability to nurse is an individual quality of those who have prepared themselves through formal education and deliberate training to help others through nursing. Nurses and other health professionals are necessary for the very existence of health service institutions. Downgrading or nonavailability of health care results when health service institutions and agencies eliminate qualified nurses and other professionals. The absence of professionally qualified public (or community) health nurses in some community health service organizations is one example of this.

Areas of Expertise and Limitations

Defining nursing practice along the eight dimensions identifies the conditions under which the nurse will be practicing nursing. A nurse's decisions about what he or she realistically can do is a first step in the regulation of the conditions under which the nurse will undertake to serve society through the practice of nursing. A second step in the regulation of practice is a nurse's examination of his or her capabilities for providing nursing to specific nursing populations. This step includes identification of areas of expertise and areas of limited knowledge, skill, and judgment where nursing consultation and supervision may be required.

Nurses and other professionals must be continuously aware of the relationship between what they know and what they do within their practice domains. Each nurse who is achieving professional standing in practice should be aware of what he or she knows and does not know, what he or she is qualified and not qualified to do in nursing, when to seek and take consultation and direction from nurses with specialized knowledge and skills, and when to coordinate nursing actions with the actions of other health workers. The nurse who is achieving professional status continues to learn to be self-directing; the professional knows what to do and what not to do and does not want, and should not need, continuous direction. Persons who aspire to function at a technical level of nursing practice should learn to expect and to insist upon the availability of professionals who will lay out the purpose and the general design of the work to be done.

Direction of Developments

A third aspect of a nurse's description and regulation of conditions of nursing practice involves identifying directions for self-development in nursing practice. The suggested desirable nurse characteristics given in Chapter 5 (see pp. 104–107) can serve nurses as one tool for self-evaluation by identifying the kinds of social, interpersonal, and technological developments that should be beneficial to them. The importance of nurses' self-regulation should not be minimized. This regulation requires that nurses understand the component elements of their capabilities to nurse (nursing agency). Unless individual nurses begin to ask and answer questions about their own nursing capabilities and to guide their developments as nurses, nursing will not progress.

One aspect of development is to consider early in a nursing career the possible practice specialties and to make judgments and decisions in light of personal interests and talents, social need, and the state of the art and science(s) of particular specialties. Specializing according to nursing populations served is or should be a matter of interest and importance to nurses. Initially nurses followed the medical pattern of specialization of practice. This pattern resulted from the use of three factors as organizing principles, namely, form of medical treatment (medical, meaning nonsurgical and surgical forms), age of patients, and body systems affected. The physician who engages in the general practice of medicine does not restrict practice by age of patients or form of treatment or part of the body affected. Usually general practitioners are restricted in their privileges to perform surgery and other highly specialized forms of medical therapy. Medical specialization has been extended to include the community and family as specialty areas.

The traditional forms of nursing specialization included medical, surgical, medical-surgical, pediatric, obstetric or maternity, maternal-infant, psychiatric–mental health, and public health or community health nursing.

Under this system of specialization, a nurse employed in a hospital in the position of staff nurse was usually expected to be equally competent in all but the last two forms of specialization. Traditionally, the practice of public health nursing included a family and neighborhood focus as well as a focus on the larger community. With changes in health care needs, with the increased recognitions of the responsibilities of individuals for their own health care, and with changes in the form and purposes of health care organizations, new specializations have emerged in nursing as well as in medicine. These include ambulatory care, long- and short-term care, care for acutely ill and chronically ill persons, and care for persons in the terminal stages of illness.

Some nurses today are preparing themselves and are practicing within a domain formed by the merging of two fields, for example, nursing and midwifery. The nurse-midwife in the United States combines the practice of nursing and the practice of midwifery in providing care for mothers, infants, and families. Other ways in which nurses are combining fields are less clear-cut. For example, some nurses who have acquired expertise in performing some aspects of medical diagnosis and treatment function primarily as physician assistants; others combine the practice of nursing and the limited practice of medicine in giving primary care within organizations where patients have access to physicians and physicians' assistants as well as nurses.

SOCIAL, INTERPERSONAL, AND TECHNOLOGICAL
DIMENSIONS OF PRACTICE

Nursing considered as a health service involves interpersonal processes since it requires the social encounter of nurses with patients and involves transactions between them. From the perspective of nurses and patients, nursing involves an "I-you" relationship. The way in which nurse and patient view "the self" and "the other" will affect what they think, feel, say, and do during their encounters. The social encounter between a nurse and a patient may last from a few minutes to days, weeks, or years. The effects of the interpersonal relationship can be far-reaching. Each may be deeply affected by his or her experiences within the health care setting.

Nurses should be guided by the knowledge that all persons are affected by their interpersonal relationships and by their membership in social groups. The functioning of two or more persons as a group is affected by the personality characteristics of the group members, their behaviors, and their relationships within and outside the group. *Group* is used here in the sense of an assemblage of persons who are related in some way and who for some time period are in communication and comparatively segregated from others.

Nurses provide nursing to individuals and to multiperson units such as families, residence groups, and special purpose groups (e.g., prenatal care groups). In nursing a number of individuals with the same type of self-care requisites, nurses may bring these persons together in groups, using the group as a method for helping individuals learn and become more able to engage in self-care. The relationships among patients and relationships among family or residence group members may be either beneficial or harmful to those involved.

Nurses approach, communicate, interact with, and provide care for persons who are in patient relationships to them, with the understanding that the relationships exist for nursing purposes. Ideally, the nurse and the patient, when the patient is able, contribute to the establishment and maintenance of an interpersonal relationship that enables each one to identify, understand, and perform essential health care and related activities according to his or her respective role in the health care situation. Ideally, nurses conduct themselves in a manner that reflects a blending of the contractual, interpersonal, and technological features of nursing practice. Table 8-1 presents these features in a summary form.

Nursing students are sometimes advised that their role as nurse is to "provide care for the whole person." This advice may be confusing or misleading when students are not helped to distinguish between nursing individuals and meeting their nonnursing needs. The position of nurse specifies that the person filling the position has a helping relationship to a patient because of the legitimate nursing needs of the patient. In providing

Table 8-1   Three Dimensions of Nursing Practice

Features	Elements		Type of relationship
	Person(s)	Person(s)	
Social	In position of *nurse* who can legitimately enter into negotiations for providng nursing	In the position of becoming a nurse's patient	Contractual for nursing
Interpersonal	*Active role* as person who is qualified and functioning as nurse	*Active role* to *no instrumental role* as person who is, was, or can be his or her own self-care agent	Professional, helping, nursing
Technological	*Nurse role set* defined by (1) the work operations of professionals and (2) the presence of a self-care deficit in the patient, including extent and causes	*Patient role set* as defined by (1) the process of diagnosis to determine needs for nursing assistance and (2) the presence and characteristics of an identified and described self-care deficit	Nursing as specified by role sets of patient and nurse

nursing within interpersonal situations to patients and members of their families, patients' needs other than nursing needs may be identified and may require consideration by the nurse. The nurse may identify the importance to the patient of finding ways to meet other needs. What the nurse does to help a patient varies with the nature of the need, legitimate ways of providing help, and the understanding and abilities of the nurse.

Ideally, the interpersonal relationship between a nurse and a patient contributes to the alleviation of the patient's stress and that of the family, enabling the patient and the family to act responsibly in matters of health and health care. A relationship that permits a patient to develop and maintain confidence in the nurse and in himself or herself is the foundation for a deliberate process of nursing that contributes positively to the patient's achievement of present and future health goals.[1]

---

[1]*The Dynamic Nurse-Patient Relationship,* by Ida Jean Orlando, G. P. Putnam's Sons, New York, 1961, and *Clinical Nursing, A Helping Art,* by Ernestine Wiedenbach, Springer, New York, 1964, focus on behavior of nurse and patient during the nursing process. "The Nature of a Science of Nursing," *Nursing Outlook,* vol. 59, May 1959, pp. 291–294, and "A Philosophy of Nursing," *Nursing Outlook,* vol. 59, April 1959, pp. 198–200, by Dorothy Johnson, indicate the nurse's role in alleviation of the patient's stress.

Some members of the health professions have expended and continue to expend effort to identify, describe, and establish the validity and reliability of approaches for working with families and other multiperson units. Some of their insights are expressed as (1) concepts of wholes, the parts of which have existence and operations apart from the whole as such, (2) concepts of families and groups as generating enduring behavioral systems and relationships, (3) concepts of formal and informal units of organization, and (4) theories of groups and group processes. In the search for valid ways to provide health care to families and other multiperson units, it has been recognized that it may be essential to work with all members of the unit in face-to-face situations, with smaller units of the larger groups, and with unit members as individuals. Providing health care to multiperson units requires the use of specialized technologies of communication, information gathering, and information processing as well as specialized regulatory technologies. Nurses who aspire to this form of practice require specialized knowledge and skills and training and the expertise necessary to help and to avoid harm for the group or its members.

THE NURSING PROCESS

Nursing is more than simply a combination of all the activities a nurse performs in behalf of a person under nursing care. For activities to be considered in the realm of nursing, they must be consciously selected and directed by the nurse toward accomplishing nursing goals within a health care situation. On this basis, the results that nurses achieve through their nursing acts are beneficial to patients to the degree that (1) the patient's therapeutic self-care is accomplished; (2) the nursing actions are helpful in moving the patient toward responsible action in matters of self-care (the patient may move toward steadily increasing independence or adapt to interruptions in the exercise of self-care capabilities or to steadily declining capacities for self-care action); or (3) members of the patient's family or a nonnurse who attends the patient become increasingly competent in making decisions relative to the continuing daily, personalized care of the patient or in providing and managing the patient's care using nurse supervision and consultation as required. One or all of these general goals of nursing action may be appropriate in specific nursing situations. Appropriateness of the general goals of nursing in specific nursing situations varies with the therapeutic self-care demand and self-care agency of the patient. How can a nurse be assured that the nursing actions she or he selects and performs in some sequential relationship will be cumulatively beneficial for the patient?

Nurses who recognize that they must have foresight in selecting the most appropriate nursing actions for their patients can have this assurance.

The necessary foresight may be acquired by systematically determining why a person requires nursing. This information, after analysis and interpretation appropriate for obtaining a nursing perspective, enables the nurse to make judgments about the characteristics of the nursing care that will make a therapeutic contribution to the patient's achievement of health and self-care goals.

Information about why a person needs nursing and a nurse's judgment about the kind of nursing required are the framework for designing a system of nursing assistance. The initial design may require modification or major revision, but throughout it remains the instrument that guides the nurse in role fulfillment. For example, if the nursing design specified a partly compensatory system of nursing with a health focus on recovery, the required universal, developmental, and health-deviation self-care components would have to be distributed to either nurse or patient for performance. For each component distributed to the patient, the nurse must specify whether the patient needs help in the form of guidance, support, or resources. For example, a patient may be able to walk and take needed exercise if a walker is provided. A sound plan would also contain details about time and place for the performance of nurse and patient activities. The nursing design provides a guide (1) to keep the actions performed by the nurse and patient in line with the nursing goals sought and (2) to maintain essential coordination between the nurse and patient and others in light of the defined roles of each in the health care situation.

A designed system of nursing assistance and the nursing plan to implement it are the results of the nurse's deliberate efforts to identify how a patient can be effectively nursed with some degree of efficiency in particular environmental setting(s). The nursing plan (or some detail of it) is the starting point for the primarily practical phase of the nursing process in which the patient (or family) is assisted in self-care matters to achieve identified and described health and health-related results. The primarily practical phase of nursing also includes (1) checking what was done against what was specified to be done, (2) collecting evidence to describe the results of care, and (3) the use of this evidence in evaluating results achieved against results specified in the nursing system design.

Determining why a person needs nursing, designing a system of nursing assistance, planning for the delivery of the specified nursing assistance, and providing and controlling the delivery of nursing assistance are referred to as the nursing process. The nursing process has its base in the theory that action to accomplish defined and limited goals must be designed and planned in relation to the goals sought; must consider the environmental, technological, and human factors relevant to goal accomplishments; must be performed according to the design, making adjustments and revisions as indicated by changing conditions; and must be controlled by evidence that the goal is being achieved, has been achieved, or is not being achieved.

The steps of the nursing process may be summarized as follows:

Step 1: The initial and continuing determination of why a person should be under nursing care.

Step 2: The designing of a system of nursing for the patient that will effectively contribute to the patient's achievement of health goals through therapeutic self-care and to the achievement of self-care or dependent-care agency goals for patient or family. Planning for the delivery of nursing according to the designed system includes specifications for roles, resources, coordinating activities, and time, place, and frequency of performance of activities by nurse, patient, or others.

Step 3: The initiation, conduction, and control of assisting actions to (1) compensate for the patient's self-care limitations to ensure that self-care is given and is therapeutic and to enable the patient to adapt his or her behavior to existing limitations, (2) overcome when possible self-care limitations of the patient (or care limitations of the family) so that the patient's future short-term or long-term therapeutic self-care requisites can be met effectively, and (3) foster and protect the patient's self-care abilities and prevent the development of new self-care limitations.

These three steps of the nursing process should be qualified as the steps of the technological component of the nursing process. In nursing, it has become customary to refer to the diagnostic, prescriptive, and regulatory operations of nursing practice as the nursing process, but these technological operations include managerial operations (e.g., planning operations) and must be coordinated with interpersonal and social processes within nursing situations. The reader should keep in mind that the steps of the nursing process as described here or elsewhere do not constitute the whole of the process of nursing patients.

In nursing practice, a nurse may be responsible for either the total process or part of the process of nursing a patient. The vocationally, technically, or professionally educated nurse when functioning as an *assistant* to a nurse who bears full nursing responsibility for a patient is a *contributor* to parts of the nursing process. Each nurse must understand the extent of his or her responsibility in each nursing situation. The American Nurses' Association and the National League for Nursing have used the steps of the nursing process in describing the functions of nurses with various types of initial preparation for nursing.[2]

In the past, too little attention was given to steps 1 and 2 of the

---

[2]See the American Nurses' Association's statements of functions of nurses in various fields of nursing practice and the National League for Nursing's statements of nursing practice outcomes for graduates of initial programs of nursing education.

nursing process. In some health care settings the need for the systematic performance of the various steps of the nursing process goes unrecognized. This does not relieve the individual nurse of responsibility for the effective performance of all three steps in the nursing process. Programs of initial and continuing education for nursing practice should be or become concerned not only with nurse capabilities as related to the systematic use of the nursing process in nursing individual patients but also with enabling nurses to introduce adequate agencywide systems for designing, planning for, and delivering personalized nursing to all clients in need of nursing. Development of adequate descriptions for nursing positions in terms relevant to both the nursing process and the nursing demands of various types of health care situations is an essential step. Nurses' capabilities and therefore their roles and needs for supervision may vary from one type of nursing case to another. In health care agencies, the pertinence of the steps of the nursing process remains in relation to both the nursing of patients and the direction, guidance, and utilization of nurses.

DIAGNOSIS AND PRESCRIPTION

The first step of the nursing process is constituted from the professional operations of diagnosis and prescription. Diagnosis is an investigative operation that enables nurses to make judgments about the existing health care situation and decisions about what can and should be done. Nurses in this phase of nursing seek answers to five questions:

1   What is the patient's therapeutic self-care demand? Now? At a future time?
2   Does the patient have a deficit for engaging in self-care to meet the therapeutic self-care demand?
3   If so, what is its nature and the reasons for its existence?
4   Should the patient be helped to refrain from engagement in self-care or to protect already developed self-care capabilities for therapeutic purposes?
5   What is the patient's potential for engaging in self-care at a future time period? Increasing or deepening self-care knowledge? Learning techniques of care? Fostering willingness to engage in self-care? Effectively and consistently incorporating essential self-care measures (including new ones) into the systems of self-care and daily living?

The investigation of these questions requires that nurses have effective ways and means to secure the essential information and to determine the qualitative and quantitative adequacy of the data collected. In practice situations nurses should collect only enough information to answer the five questions.

Every situation of nursing practice is different. Nurses may be guided in nursing practice by general rules, for example, the rule that *diagnosis precedes prescription and regulation or treatment,* or the rule that *nursing diagnosis seeks answers to five questions.* However, because of the specific nature of each situation of nursing practice, it is the individual nurse who must establish how to proceed, using general or more specific rules of practice as guides in making judgments and decisions. One danger to be avoided for the protection of patients and nurses is making nursing diagnoses and prescriptions on the basis of inadequate data about patients. On the other hand, nurses can become so taken with information gathering that they lose sight of the reasons why an individual is under health care and of the usefulness of the collected information for purposes of nursing practice.

The diagnostic and prescriptive operations of nurses concerning patients' therapeutic self-care demands and self-care agency must be coordinated with interpersonal operations and the contractual operations performed with patients or with persons acting for them. These operations are identified in two sets, one related to patients' therapeutic self-care demands and the other to their existing and potential ability to engage in self-care. They are summarized in Tables 8-2 and 8-3.

The contractual nature of nurse-patient relationships requires that patients and members of their families know their existing and continuing or changing requirements for self-care and their roles and the roles of nurses and others in the continuous provision of care. If nurses would accept the purpose of nursing and the contractual nature of nursing relationships, the deleterious practices of viewing patients as objects to be acted on and of processing patients through a system of routinized measures regardless of their conditions and needs might be eliminated.

In Tables 8-2 and 8-3 the diagnostic and prescriptive operations of nursing have been made explicit as to form; they have been correlated with interpersonal and contractual operations; and the types of results of the operations have been indicated. The specification of these operations requires that nurses be constantly aware of what patients are experiencing and feeling and what help and regulatory nursing care should be provided on the basis of preliminary and cursory diagnosis. Nursing diagnosis and prescription are ongoing processes that continue as long as a person is under nursing care, but nurses perform them initially in their early contacts with patients. The health care focus of the nursing care (Chapter 6) will influence nurses' initial and subsequent approaches to the operations of nursing diagnosis and prescription.

Patient and Family Collaboration

In the first as well as in subsequent steps of the nursing process, patients' and families' abilities to and interest in collaborating with nurses affect what nurses can do. Patients, members of their families, or others who are acting for patients may or may not be interested in the need or psychologically able to accept the need for collaboration with nurses or the need for being or becoming active participants in their own self-care or the care of their dependents. For this reason, it is important for nurses to make initial observations about patients and their families in order to provide themselves with information they can use to guide their interactions and communications with patients.

From this perspective, nurses should concern themselves with (1) identifying the personality characteristics of patients and others related to them that will significantly affect the nursing situation (e.g., passivity-activity) and (2) identifying and exploring patients' concerns that may block their active collaboration with nurses and their participation in health care. To obtain this information, nurses must make observations on and elicit subjective information from patients. Nurses should also be alert to situations where patients never question what nurses say and do. It is important for nurses to know whether patients are understanding and accepting, or uninvolved, or always accepting of what persons in position of authority say, or fearful or unknowing. Such information should be limited to what is essential to know in order to work with patients and families. Patients' interests in and concern for their integrated functioning, their acceptance of the reality of their states of functioning, and their need for particular care measures will affect what patients will and will not do. Meeting the universal self-care requisite for promotion of integrated functioning and normalcy by patients is a first step toward their collaboration with nurses and their participation in self-care.

DESIGNING AND PLANNING

Designing and planning occupy a middle position in the technological nursing process. They follow diagnosis and prescription and precede the production and management of systems of nursing assistance. Designing nursing systems is a professional nursing operation, and planning their production is a management operation. The degree to which designing nursing systems and planning their production can be separately performed in a block of time in between steps one and three of the nursing process varies. Factors that militate against this include (1) rapid and complex changes in the health states of patients, (2) needs for continuous adjustments in patients' therapeutic self-care demands, (3) insufficient amounts of valid and reliable factual information about patients and their environments, and (4) inability of the nurse to predict the future values of the patient variables (therapeutic self-care demand and self-care agency). For example, when the vital functions of patients are unstable, design and planning become interspersed between the minute-to-minute decisions

Table 8-2 Operations Related to Determining Patients' Therapeutic Self-Care Demands

Interpersonal and contractual operations	Technological-professional operations			Types of operations
Entering into and maintaining effective relationships with patient, family, or significant others				
Reach an agreement (implicit or explicit) with the patient or family to seek answers to the question, What is the patient's therapeutic self-care demand at this time? In the future?				
Collaborate with patient or family	Determine the existing and projected self-care requisites, their particular values, and expected changes in their values			Diagnostic—of self-care requisites
Review with patient or family	*Existing requisites*	*Current values*	*Projected requisites*	*Projected values*
	Universal		Universal	
	Developmental		Developmental	
	Health-deviation		Health-deviation	
Collaborate with patient or family	Determine the methods through which each existing or projected self-care requisite can be met, i.e., methods that are valid and reliable in relation to the patient's age, developmental state, health state, and other conditioning factors			Preliminary—prescriptive operations
Review with patient or family	Select the methods that will be used for meeting each particularized self-care requisite, with knowledge of the safety and degree of effectiveness of each method			

	Lay out the procedures or care measures required for using the selected method(s) for meeting each of the requisites	
Review with patient or family	Calculate the ideal therapeutic self-care demand and identify self-care requisites with high priorities	Prescriptive of the ideal therapeutic self-care demand for some duration

Self-care requisites	Values	Methods	Measures for meeting
Universal			
Developmental			
Health-deviation			

Reach agreements with patient or family about the constituent parts of the therapeutic self-care demand, and give the final prescription of the therapeutic self-care demand to the patient or family	Make adjustments as required in the therapeutic self-care demand to bring it into accord with what is possible (and necessary) to accomplish	Final—prescriptive of the therapeutic self-care demand
Specify nurse, patient, or family roles in making adjustments	Identify factors that will require changes in the values of self-care requisites. Indicate how to calculate value changes and to make adjustments in methods or procedures as these are needed during time	Specification of rules for making changes in the therapeutic self-care demand

Table 8-3   Operations Related to Self-Care Agency and Its Regulation

Interpersonal and contractual operations	Technological-professional operations	Types of operation
Entering into and maintaining effective relationships with patient, family, or significant others		
Reach an agreement (implicit or explicit) to seek answers to the question, Can and to what degree can the patient engage in required self-care at this time? At a future time?		
Collaborate with patient or family	Identify and describe the patient's repertoire of self-care practices and the usual components of the patient's self-care system	Diagnostic of self-care agency
Collaborate with patient or family	Identify and describe limitations for deliberate action that interfere with the decision-making and productive phases of self-care, including medically prescribed restriction of activity	
Review conclusions with patient or family	Make inferences about the general abilities and limitations of the patient for engagement in the decision-making and productive phases of self-care; formulate and express as judgments	
	Validate inferences through continued observation of what the patient does and does not do	

Table 8-3 Operations Related to Self-Care Agency and Its Regulation
(*Continued*)

Interpersonal and contractual operations	Technological-professional operations	Types of operation
Collaborate and reach agreements with patient or family	Determine the adequacy of the patient's knowledge, skills, and willingness to meet each self-care requisite using particular methods and measures of care	
Inform patient or family of the judgment about the presence or absence of a self-care deficit	Make and express judgments about what the patient is able to do, not able to do, and what the patient should not do in meeting the prescribed therapeutic self-care demand, at this time or at a future time	Diagnostic of the presence or absence of a self-care deficit—existing; projected
Reach agreements about prescribed roles with patient or family, with nurses, or with dependent-care agents	In light of the presence and nature of a self-care deficit determine what the patient should do and should not do and what the patient is willing to do in the immediate meeting of the prescribed therapeutic self-care demand	Prescription of patient role and nurse role (or dependent-care agent role) in meeting the therapeutic self-care demand
Reach agreements with patient about prescribed patient role and related nurse role	In the event of an existing or a potential self-care deficit determine the potential for the future exercise of or the continued development of self-care agency	Prescription of patient role and related nurse role in regulating the exercise or development of self-care agency

nurses make about what they should and should not do on the basis of a continuous flow of patient information.

The scope and depth of the design of a nursing system and the plan for its production cannot exceed the amount of reliable patient information available. A nursing design may be tentative—no more than a set of day-to-day working instructions. In such situations the effective and proper design of a nursing system for a particular patient may emerge as nurses work with that patient and observe what is effective and what is not. Designs for nursing systems and plans for their production that are based upon inadequate, incomplete, or incorrect information or upon misinterpretation of the meaning of information may produce more harm than good for patients. Designing systems of nursing that should be valid for some period of time is possible whenever there is a moderate to high degree of stability in the health states of patients and their environmental situations. When a number of variations in the psychological or physiological aspects of patient functioning may occur, it is necessary to build each possible occurrence into the nursing system design.

This second step of the technological nursing process is essential in all nursing situations, regardless of the degree to which it can be separated out for performance. Whenever nursing diagnoses and prescriptions for therapeutic self-care demands and for nurse and patient roles are valid for a day or more, nurses should engage in more formal processes of design and planning. Professionally qualified nurses should understand that designing and planning are major components of their work; whenever technically educated nurses contribute to the production of nursing systems, plans should be expressed and available to them.

Nursing Systems Design

Designing nursing systems consists essentially of two operations. The first operation is bringing about a *good organization of the components of patients'* therapeutic self-care demands. The second operation is the *selection of the combination of ways of helping* that will be both effective and efficient in *compensating for or overcoming patients' self-care deficits*. The components of the therapeutic self-care demand should be related in terms of (1) time sequence of performance, (2) combined action in achieving goals related to the regulation of states of health and development, and (3) the effects that a particular course of action in meeting one self-care requisite will have on meeting other self-care requisites.

As indicated in Table 8-2 and in Chapter 3, once self-care requisites have been specified for an individual, they are met through the *performance of courses or systems of action*. These courses of action have their origins in the specific self-care requisites and in the methods for meeting them. Methods or equipment may need to be adjusted for factors such as age; for example, variations in methods of feeding infants and children set up different requirements for feeding equipment. The courses of actions to meet each self-care requisite become the work operations of self-care, the tasks to be performed. Bringing about a good organization of these tasks is the first movement toward a good nursing system design. The second movement of design is to specify who and to what degree nurses and patients will be involved in (1) the production of patients' self-care, including the maintenance of the organization of self-care tasks and (2) the regulation of the exercise or development of the patient's self-care agency.

As a result of nursing diagnosis and prescription nurses have degrees of knowledge of the presence of, extent of, and reasons for the existence of self-care deficits. They have knowledge about the instrumental role of the patient in the production and management of self-care (e.g., no role, some role). The purposes of design are (1) to create that system of relationships among the components of the therapeutic self-care demand that will result in good regulation of the health and developmental state of the patient, (2) to specify the timing and the amount of nurse-patient contact and the reasons for it, and (3) to identify the contributions of nurse and patient to meeting the therapeutic self-care demand, to making adjustments in it, and to regulating the exercise or development of self-care agency.

Certain matters should be held in mind by nurses as they design systems of nursing for patients. For example, some self-care actions, particularly those involving choice, decision, and will, cannot be performed for a patient by anyone else. The provision of appropriate support and environmental conditions may help the patient to gradually acquire competence in these matters. In relation to a patient's requirements for sleep, rest, and activity, nurses may be able to establish and maintain environmental conditions that are conducive to rest, sleep, or activity, including the control of demands placed upon the patient. Nurses should also keep in mind that patients may want to do more than they are physically or psychologically able to do. Provisions to help patients set limits on what they are to do in self-care should be included in the nursing system design. Some patients may not desire or be willing to engage in self-care even when they are able by objective standards. Here again, nurses may need to foresee the desirability of providing environmental conditions that will encourage or induce patients to assume self-care responsibility.

Patients who want to perform beyond their capacities may test themselves and learn from experience that they cannot do what they had judged themselves able to do. In the same way, reluctant or unwilling patients, when confronted by nurses who want to and know how to assist them to become self-directing, can often move quickly to engage in decision-making and planning activities relating to self-care and to perform selected self-care tasks. In both of these instances, nurses and patients are not in agreement about who shall do what. They are not cooperating in an agreed upon manner (positive cooperation); they are engaged in a struggle (negative cooperation.)[3] This type of cooperation is valid only if nurses' judgments about patients' abilities are sound and if they are motivated by a

[3]Tadeusz Kotarbinski, *Praxiology,* Pergamon Press, New York, 1965, pp. 62–64.

sincere desire to conserve patients' energies or to help them assume their self-care responsibility. Nurses must be certain, however, that the basis for action is a valid one so that the situation will not dissolve into a battle of wills. In designing a nursing system, evidence that indicates that positive or negative cooperation will prevail should be taken into consideration. Thus, an important element in designing a nursing system for a patient and in planning for the complement of nurses required is the identification of the extent and intensity of nurse-patient interaction which is required in order to meet nursing requirements. The psychological effects of nursing in various types of health care situations on nurses should be thoroughly studied as one of the principal elements for determining more effective and efficient nursing system designs.

Designing an effective and efficient system of nursing is essentially a process of selecting valid ways of assisting a patient once self-care requisites and limitations are identified and described. The immediacy of patients' needs for self-care, as well as the nature of their self-care limitations, may affect nurses' choices of ways of assisting patients. The nurse uses two types of knowledge in order to design valid nursing systems for patients. One type of knowledge is factual and is derived from or related to the patient. It describes the patient from a nursing perspective and includes detailed descriptions of his or her abilities and limitations for self-care. This information is acquired and organized through activities that were described in step 1 of the nursing process. The other type of knowledge is general and relates to accumulated information about types of therapeutic self-care demands and how the ways of helping can compensate for or overcome limitations for therapeutic self-care. It takes into account the health-related causes of these conditions and factors that affect the effective use of the ways of helping.

When what a nurse will do and what a patient will do in relation to the patient's self-care and in adapting to, compensating for, or overcoming self-care limitations are determined by the selected ways of assisting, a pattern or design of a system emerges. The design of a nursing system for a specific patient will be more detailed in that the roles of nurse and patient will be described in relation to (1) self-care tasks to be performed in coordinated patterns and in particular time sequences, (2) making adjustments in the therapeutic self-care demands, (3) regulating the exercise of self-care agency, (4) protecting developed powers of self-care agency, and (5) bringing about new development in self-care agency (e.g., acquiring knowledge, developing specific skills).

In making decisions about how to help patients effectively extend their self-care capabilities, it is necessary for a nurse to have for recall a body of knowledge about self-care as deliberate action. Understanding based on previously presented information about the conditions essential for self-care (Chapter 5) may be extended by a further consideration of the concept that some self-care behaviors are internally oriented and others are externally oriented.

The internally oriented behaviors required for self-care are:

1 Learning activities related to the development of self-care knowledge, attitudes, and skills
2 Application of knowledge in initiating, performing, and controlling self-care activities
3 Self-care action to control behavior, such as controlling an emotional reaction, facing the reality of one's state of health or disability, or restricting one's activities in order to rest or to keep a part of the body immobilized
4 Action to monitor one's condition or responses

The externally oriented behaviors required for self-care are:

1 Knowledge-seeking activity directed to printed material or to persons who possess knowledge about health, disease, and effective self-care practices
2 Resource-seeking activity related to securing equipment, materials, facilities, and services necessary in self-care
3 Resource-utilizing activities related to using supplies or equipment in performing self-care
4 Activity to control factors in the external environment, for example, controlling the movement of air, the number of social contacts, or biological elements in the environment
5 Activity to seek assistance to accomplish a self-care goal within an interpersonal situation, for example, requesting help in performing a self-care task, seeking validation of a judgment, or asking not to be left alone
6 Expressive interpersonal activity, such as when a patient expresses feelings about health or self-care verbally or nonverbally but without a direct request for help
7 Action to become aware of one's location in an environment or of environmental conditions[4]

The internally oriented behaviors necessary in self-care are behaviors that are dependent upon awareness of self and environment, as well as upon motivation and interest. The internally oriented self-care behaviors of a patient at any particular time are always dependent in part upon

[4]This revised listing of types of self-care behaviors was originally developed by the author. It was reviewed and revised by members of a faculty committee, the Committee on the Nursing Model, School of Nursing, Catholic University of America, Washington, D.C., in 1966–1967. See Fig. 4-2, which indicates the directional flow of some of these behaviors.

acquired knowledge about the goals and practices of self-care. This knowledge may have been acquired in the family setting, in school, in social contacts with friends and associates, or through previous contacts with physicians and other health workers. The presence of limitations in awareness, in valid knowledge about the nature and meaning of self-care, in self-care skills, and in initiating, directing, and controlling behavior to accomplish defined goals of self-care affect a patient's internally oriented self-care behavior.

The externally oriented self-care behaviors are need-fulfilling behaviors with an external environmental orientation. Factors in the patient or in the environment may be instrumental in prompting a person to behave in one of these ways. Ability to engage in specific goal-seeking activities is a prerequisite for externally oriented self-care behaviors 1 to 7. In a nursing situation, the kinds of externally oriented behaviors in which a patient will seek to engage or should be helped to engage are related to the patient's self-care habits, perceived needs for care, objective requirements for care, and need to express feelings or impart or secure information. Environmental conditions as well as the person's capacity for various forms of deliberate action are relevant to these behaviors.

In summary, the nurse's knowledge of the patient's (1) objective requirements for therapeutic self-care now and in the future when related to the patient's (2) interests in, desire for, and concerns about self-care, and (3) immediate and projected future capacities and limitations for self-care enable the nurse to (4) make judgments about appropriate ways of helping the patient to (5) provide therapeutic self-care and (6) accomplish appropriate self-care agency goals. Thus an effective nursing system provides ways of relating the behaviors of both nurse and patient to the accomplishment of nursing goals appropriate to the situation. Adjustment of nurse and patient behaviors to immediate conditions and to projected future conditions is accomplished through the selection of helping methods and definition of roles (Chapters 4 and 5). The nature of the patient's specific limitations for self-care and the patient's degree of deficit for self-care are important considerations, as is the health care focus.

When a nurse selects a system of assistance for the immediate care of a patient, he or she may not have sufficient knowledge for making projections about how the selected forms of assistance should change with anticipated changes in the patient's condition. Nurses should systematically collect information about their patients to enable them to project requirements for changes in the initially selected system. Designing systems of nursing assistance for individual patients is not a common activity of nurses in health care agencies. Designing is an essential nursing activity, since a nursing plan has as its central focus the delivery of some selected system of nursing assistance.

Planning

Planning as an aspect of the technological nursing process is the further development of designs for nursing systems or for portions of such systems. A design for a nursing system is essentially a plan in broad relief—a plan that sets forth the organization and timing of essential tasks to be performed, allocates their performance to nurse or patient, and designates how patients are to be helped by nurses in task performance. If a design is a partial one, the plan for using the design to guide nursing actions will also be a partial one. *Partial* is used in the sense of not complete, related to the duration of time that a person will be under nursing care. At times, nurses may not separate design and planning operations from diagnostic and prescriptive operations. In such instances plans are short-term and are integrated with nurses' judgments and decisions about the specific task performance of nurses and patients.

Planning adds to the proposed nursing system specifications of the time, place, environmental conditions, and equipment and supplies required for the production of the system. Planning also produces specifications for the number and the qualifications of nurses or others necessary in order to produce a designed nursing system or a portion thereof, to evaluate effects, and to make needed adjustments. When planning is for the performance of a selected self-care task, it may amount to a judgment by a nurse that, under prevailing conditions, the nurse will take this action here and now for the well-being of the patient, for example, "The patient can and should do this. I will remain here to support the patient. Betty will get the supplies needed." In scheduling the performance of self-care measures nurses should take into consideration (1) the relationships among the components of a patient's therapeutic self-care demands, for example, arranging the performance of measures of self-care to enable patients to have periods of uninterrupted rest and sleep and (2) the provision for assistance when patients need it, for example, in helping patients with elimination.

PRODUCING CARE TO REGULATE THERAPEUTIC SELF-CARE DEMAND AND SELF-CARE AGENCY

Regulatory nursing systems are produced when nurses interact with patients and take consistent action to meet their prescribed therapeutic self-care demands and to regulate the exercise or development of their capabilities for self-care. A valid design for one or for a series of nursing systems to be instituted for a patient can be used as a guide in the production and management of nursing systems. The planning for implementation of the design and related procurement activities will determine if nurses can be with patients and if essential materials and equipment will be available and in readiness for use. In this, the third step of the technological nursing process, nurses act to help patients meet their therapeutic self-care demands and regulate the exercise or development of their abilities to engage in self-care.

Systems of nursing oriented to regulation or treatment should be produced and managed for patients as long as the self-care or dependent-care deficits exist. Systems of regulatory nursing at times are replaced by systems of assistance provided by persons other than the nurse who are prepared to perform some measures of self-care for others. In such instances, nursing consultation and supervision should be available to both the person with the care deficit and the persons who are providing care. In all such situations, a professional nurse should participate in the development of the care system design whenever patients and families are unable to do this.

Regulatory nursing systems are produced through the actions of nurses and their patients during nurse-patient encounters. Nurses during these encounters will take action to:

1 Perform and regulate the self-care tasks for patients or assist patients with their performance of self-care tasks

2 Coordinate self-care task performance so that a unified system of care is produced and coordinated with other components of health care

3 Help patients, their families, and others bring about systems of daily living for patients that support the accomplishment of self-care and are, at the same time, satisfying in relation to patients' interest, talents, and goals

4 Guide, direct, and support patients in their exercise of, or in withholding the exercise of, their self-care agency

5 Stimulate patients' interest in self-care by raising questions and promoting discussions of care problems and issues when conditions permit

6 Support and guide patients in learning activities and provide cues for learning as well as instructional sessions

7 Support and guide patients as they experience illness or disability and the effects of medical care measures and as they experience the need to engage in new measures of self-care or change their ways of meeting ongoing self-care requisites

8 Monitor patients and assist patients to monitor themselves to determine if self-care measures were performed and to determine the effects of self-care, the results of efforts to regulate the exercise or development of self-care agency, and the sufficiency and efficiency of nursing action directed to these ends

9 Make characterizing judgments about the sufficiency and efficiency of self-care, the regulation of the exercise or development of self-care agency, and nursing assistance

10 Make judgments about the meaning of the results derived from nurses' performance of 8 and 9 for the well-being of patients and make or recommend adjustments in the nursing care system through changes in nurse and patient roles

Operations 1 through 7 constitute direct nursing care, that is, the action system that makes up the treatment or the regulatory phase of nursing. These operations are performed by nurses at moments when patients can benefit from these seven operations. They are selected and performed by nurses in accordance with the presenting needs and conditions of patients. Operations 8, 9, and 10 are for the purpose of deciding if direct nursing care should be continued in the present form or if it should be changed. Nurses' performance of operations 1 through 7 and facts about patients' presenting needs and conditions are recorded in patients' charts to document nurses' day-to-day direct care, treatment, or actions. The results and recommendations resulting from nurses' performance of operations 8 to 10 are recorded as progress notations. Such notations document the basis for nurses' judgments about the effects of patients' current self-care regimens and care systems and the sufficiency and efficiency of nursing.

The direct nursing care actions of nurses may be started during nurses' first encounters with patients during the period of initial nursing diagnosis. Assisting patients with self-care or performing some parts of the other direct care operations cannot be deferred until nursing diagnosis is complete or until there is a formalized design for a regulatory nursing system. Diagnostic, prescriptive, and design and planning operations may be sequentially performed in relation to direct care actions.

To understand the production of regulatory nursing care it is necessary to visualize the distribution and duration of nurse-patient encounters, the kinds of operations nurses engage in during these encounters, the nursing focus maintained by nurses in relation to known health care focuses, and the helping methods nurses select in relation to the presenting needs and conditions of the patient and existing environmental conditions. The need for the performance of some self-care tasks at particular times can be anticipated. The degree to which tasks to meet patients' therapeutic self-care demands and to regulate self-care agency can be programmed by time and place varies with the stability of patients' health states and their health care regimens. The number of nurses required to produce a system of nursing for a patient varies with the intermittent or continuous nature of patients' self-care requisites; degrees of physical helplessness and dependency on others; states of development; the degree of stability of health states; the familiarity or strangeness of the environments in which health care is received; and, of course, what individual nurses can do and should do within a particular time period. The frequency and duration of contact between nurse and patient must be sufficient for the intermittent or continuous performance of some or all of the ten operations required for the production of effective regulatory nursing care systems.

Nursing practice situations where patients require nursing over the 24 hours of the day range from those where a professionally qualified nurse is unable or just able to provide continuous nursing for one patient without assistance to those where one nurse can effectively provide care to a number of patients during the same time period with or without assistance. In ambulatory care, nurses may carry large case loads of patients, the number of patients being related to the frequency of required nurse-patient contacts and the length of visits. When nursing is provided through home visits by the nurse, the number of patients in a nurse's case load is affected by the frequency of visits, the kind and amount of care provided, and travel time. When more than one nurse is contributing to the production of nursing assistance, there are requirements for coordinating nursing operations, clarifying the goals being sought through nursing, and socializing patients to a number of nurses. In a situation of this type, patients are often unaware of their own roles and the roles of nurses with whom they have contact.

Nursing Service in the Community

Many communities in the United States and elsewhere expect nursing to be available on a communitywide basis. The pattern for nursing as a community service to individuals and families was set in the United States during the latter part of the nineteenth century. One type of nursing focused on caring for the sick or disabled in their homes and instructing the family in hygiene and sanitation measures.[5] This type of nursing was known as *district nursing*. It was provided by nurses employed by district or local health service agencies.

Another type of nursing was the care of the sick in their homes by nurses who were employed by patients or their families. This type of nursing was known as *private-duty nursing*. A third type of nursing was caring for the sick in hospitals or other institutions. This was known as *hospital* or *institutional nursing*.[6] The pattern for nursing in communities has changed since the developmental years, but modern nursing practice can be traced back to these three types of nursing service.

What quality and quantity of nursing service are available to a modern community? What are the costs involved in providing this service to the community? What must patients pay for nursing, and how and where can

[5]Isabel A. Hampton, et al., *Nursing of the Sick 1893*, McGraw-Hill, New York, 1949, pp. 119–136.
[6]Ibid., pp. 191–201.

they obtain this assistance when it is required? These are important questions that must be answered, partly by the citizens of the community and partly by nurses. Nursing, like the other services established in a community for the health, welfare, and safety of its citizens, must be planned for, maintained, and developed in keeping with community needs. If a community is to have nursing available, it must have nurses, and each community, therefore, must answer the question, "How can this community fulfill its needs for nurses?"

The strength and effectiveness of nursing as a health service in the community depends upon the values of the community. The provision of nursing makes heavy demands on community resources. Many persons in a community need nursing at the same time—in their homes, in hospitals and clinics, in nursing homes and homes for the aged, in child-care institutions and clinics, and in a variety of other facilities providing health service. A community may require large numbers of nurses to supply the demands for nursing that exist at the same time, and often in the same place, throughout the 24 hours of each day and each day throughout the year. From both the community's point of view and the patient's point of view, nursing is a costly service and one that frequently may be in short supply. A community that is convinced that nursing is an essential health service will be more likely to engage in activities and programs necessary for providing adequate nursing service than will the community that holds no such conviction. In addition, many communities face the problem of finding candidates for nursing careers and preparing them for nursing practice.

The types of nurses needed and the educational facilities available for preparation for nursing practice are also factors that must be considered in providing adequate nursing in the community. Before World War II, nurses were educated almost exclusively in schools maintained and controlled by local hospitals. The level of preparation for all nursing personnel was essentially the same. Since that time, the increasing demand for nurses, the shortage of nurses, and the increasing complexity of health care has resulted in the preparation of persons for work in nursing in all the existing forms of occupational education and training. The number and the qualifications of persons employed to provide nursing often differ from the required number of nurses who are qualified to give nursing.

Nurses' failure to develop or implement standards of nursing practice in the community has resulted at times in ineffective nursing and undesirable conditions of practice. Licensed nurses may not be prepared, able, or willing to design, provide, and manage systems of nursing assistance for patients and to supervise other nurses and auxiliary workers who contribute to the daily provision of nursing for individuals. Nurses often are not present or are so infrequently or remotely available that patients have little or no contact with them. As a result, technically prepared nurses, practical nurses, and nursing aides are placed in positions they are unprepared to fill.

The growing interest of the American Nurses' Association in the development and implementation of standards of nursing practice to enhance the quality of nursing provided in community health agencies and hospitals should bring about improved conditions for both the consumers and practitioners of nursing.

The development of criterion measures of nursing care along with instruments and procedures for use in measuring the quality of nursing provided in a health care facility is making an important contribution to nursing. The work of Barbara J. Horn and Mary Ann Swain and their associates (see Selected Readings) is an example of such work. In this project, criterion measures were developed around the universal self-care requisites and health-deviation self-care requisites. Continued effort to ensure that the nursing provided in particular settings is in accord with patients' self-care deficits is needed. This effort, however, should be accompanied by efforts to provide qualified nurses with opportunities to engage in nursing diagnosis and prescription and in the design, production, and management of effective nursing systems for individuals and groups.

SELECTED READINGS

Allison, S. E.: "A Framework for Nursing Action in a Nurse Conducted Diabetic Management Clinic," *Journal of Nursing Administration*, vol. 3, July-August 1973, pp. 53–60.

Backscheider, J. E.: "The Use of Self as the Essence of Clinical Supervision in Ambulatory Patient Care," *Nursing Clinics of North America*, vol. 6, December 1971, pp. 785–794.

Casoly, Rose Marie: "Give the Patient His Due," *American Journal of Nursing*, vol. 72, June 1972, p. 1101.

Conant, Lucy H.: "Give and Take in Home Visits," *American Journal of Nursing*, vol. 65, July 1965, pp. 117–120.

Doughty, Dorothy Beckley, and Norma Justus Mash: *Nursing Audit*, F. A. Davis, Philadelphia, 1977.

Gergen, Kenneth J.: "The Significance of Skin Color in Human Relations," *Daedalus*, Spring 1967, pp. 390–406.

Griffin, Winnie, Sara J. Anderson, and Joyce Y. Passos: "Group Exercises for Patients with Limited Motion," *American Journal of Nursing*, vol. 71, September 1971, pp. 42–43.

Horn, Barbara J., and Mary Ann Swain: *Development of Criterion Measures of Nursing Care, vols. 1 and 2*, University of Michigan and National Center for Health Services Research, U.S. Department of Commerce, National Technical Information Service, Springfield, Va., 1978. Publication nos. 267-004 and 267-005.

Jonas, Steven: "Limitations of Community Control of Health Facilities and Services: An Editorial," *American Journal of Public Health,* vol. 68, June 1978, pp. 541–543.

Larson, Sister Paula A.: "Influence of Patient Status and Health Condition on Nurse Perceptions of Patient Characteristics," *Nursing Research,* vol. 26, November-December 1977, pp. 416–421.

Lenarz, Dorothea M.: "Caring Is the Essence of Practice," *American Journal of Nursing,* vol. 71, April 1971, pp. 704–707.

Meyer, Rita M. Sczekalla, and Diane Torzewski Morris: "Alcoholic Cardiomyopathy: A Nursing Approach," *Nursing Research,* vol. 26, November-December 1977, pp. 422–427.

Pesznecker, Betty L., and Mary Ann Droye: "Family Nurse Practitioners in Primary Care: A Study of Practice and Patients," *American Journal of Public Health,* vol. 68, October 1978, pp. 977–980. ,

Schwartz, Doris, et al.: "Problems of Ambulation and Traveling among Elderly, Chronically Ill Clinic Patients," *Nursing Research,* vol. 12, Summer 1963, pp. 165–171.

Serafini, Patricia: "Nursing Assessment in Industry," *American Journal of Public Health,* vol. 66, August 1976, pp. 755–760.

Sullivan, Judith A., et al.: "The Rural Nurse Practitioner: A Challenge and a Response," *American Journal of Public Health,* vol. 68, October 1978, pp. 972–976.

Travelbee, Joyce: "What's Wrong with Sympathy?" *American Journal of Nursing,* vol. 64, January 1964, pp. 68–71.

Bibliography

Ackerman, Nathan W.: *The Psychodynamics of Family Life*, Basic Books, Inc., New York, 1958.

Allison, Sarah E.: *The Meaning of Rest: Some Views and Behaviors Characterizing Rest as a State and a Process, An Exploratory Nursing Study*, doctoral dissertation, Teachers' College, Columbia University, New York, 1968.

Allport, Gordon W.: *Becoming: Basic Considerations for a Psychology of Personality*, Yale University Press, New Haven, 1955.

———: *Personality and Social Encounter: Selected Essays*, Beacon Press, Boston, 1960.

———: *Pattern and Growth in Personality*, Holt, Rinehart and Winston, New York, 1965.

Andersen, Ronald, and Odin Anderson: *A Decade of Health Services: Social Survey Trends in Use and Expenditure*, University of Chicago Press, Chicago, 1967.

Arnold, Magda B.: *Emotion and Personality*, vol. 1: *Psychological Aspects*, Columbia University Press, New York, 1960.

———: *Emotion and Personality*, vol. 2: *Neurological and Physiological Aspects*, Columbia University Press, New York, 1960.

Ashby, W. Ross: *An Introduction to Cybernetics*, Chapman & Hall Ltd., London, 1964.

Barnard, Chester I.: *The Functions of the Executive*, Harvard University Press, Cambridge, Mass., 1962.

Blocker, Clyde E., Robert H. Plummer, and Richard C. Richardson, Jr.: *The Two-Year College: A Social Synthesis*, Prentice-Hall, Englewood Cliffs, N.J., 1965.

Brooks, Dorothy Lee: *Identification of Selected Nursing Factors to Determine the Availability of Learning Experiences for Students*, master's thesis, School of Nursing, Catholic University of America, Washington, D.C., 1963.

Buckley, Walter: *Sociology and Modern Systems Theory*, Prentice-Hall, Englewood Cliffs, N.J., 1967.

Dubos, René: "Humanistic Biology," *American Scholar*, vol. 34, Spring 1965, pp. 179–198.

————: *Man Adapting*, Yale University Press, New Haven, 1965.

Entralgo, P. Lain: *Doctor and Patient*, Frances Partridge (trans.), World University Library, McGraw-Hill, New York, 1969.

Firth, Raymond: *Elements of Social Organization*, 3d ed., Beacon Press, Boston, 1961.

Foucault, Michel: *The Birth of the Clinic: An Archaeology of Medical Perception*, A. M. Sheridan Smith (trans.), Vintage Books, New York, 1975.

Fromm, Erich: *The Heart of Man*, Harper & Row, New York, 1968.

Galdston, Iago: *Medicine in Transition*, University of Chicago Press, Chicago, 1965.

Hall, Lydia E.: "Another View of Nursing Care and Quality," in K. M. Straub and Kitty S. Parker (eds.), *Continuity of Patient Care: The Role of Nursing*, Catholic University of America Press, Washington, D.C., 1966, pp. 47–60.

Hampton, Isabel A., et al.: *Nursing of the Sick 1893*, McGraw-Hill, New York, 1949.

Harrison, T. R., et al. (eds.): *Principles of Internal Medicine*, 5th ed., McGraw-Hill, New York, 1966.

Hartnett, Sister Louise Marie: *Development of a Theoretical Model for the Identification of Nursing Requirements in a Selected Aspect of Self-Care*, master's thesis, School of Nursing, Catholic University of America, Washington, D.C., 1968.

Helson, Harry: *Adaptation-Level Theory: An Experimental and Systematic Approach to Behavior*, Harper & Row, New York, 1964.

Henderson, Virginia: *The Nature of Nursing: A Definition and Its Implications for Practice, Research, and Education*, Macmillan, New York, 1966.

Houssay, Bernardo A., et al.: *Human Physiology*, McGraw-Hill, New York, 1955.

Illich, Ivan: *Medical Nemesis*, Pantheon Books, New York, 1976.

Jaco, E. Gartly (ed.): *Patients, Physicians and Illness: Sourcebook in Behavioral Science and Medicine*, Free Press, Glencoe, Ill., 1958.

Johns, Edward B., Wilfred C. Sutton, and Lloyd E. Webster: *Health for Effective Living*, 3d ed., McGraw-Hill, New York, 1962, pp. 282–286.

Katz, Robert L.: *Empathy, Its Nature and Uses*, Free Press, New York, 1963.

Knutson, Andie L.: *The Individual, Society, and Health Behavior,* Russell Sage Foundation, New York, 1965.

Kotarbinski, Taduesz: *Praxiology: An Introduction to the Sciences of Efficient Action,* Olgierd Wojtasiewicz (trans.), 1st English ed., Pergamon Press, New York, 1965.

Leavell, Hugh Rodman, and E. Gurney Clark, et al.: *Preventive Medicine for the Doctor in His Community,* 3d ed., McGraw-Hill, New York, 1965.

Lewin, Kurt: *Field Theory in Social Science, Selected Theoretical Papers,* Dorwin Cartwright (ed.), Harper Torchbooks, New York, 1951.

Lonergan, Bernard J. F.: *Insight, A Study of Human Understanding,* Philosophical Library, New York, 1958.

McHale, John: "Global Ecology: Toward the Planetary Society," *American Behavioral Scientist,* vol. 11, July-August 1968, pp. 29–33.

Macmurray, John: *The Self as Agent,* Faber and Faber, London, 1957.

Mechanic, David: *Medical Sociology: A Selective View,* Free Press, New York, 1968.

Monnig, Sister M. Gretta: *Identification and Description of Nursing Opportunities for Health Teaching of Patients with Gastric Surgery as a Basis for Curriculum Development in Nursing,* master's thesis, School of Nursing, Catholic University of America, Washington, D.C., 1965.

Nadel, S. F.: *The Theory of Social Structure,* Free Press, Glencoe, Ill., 1958.

Nagel, Ernest: *The Structure of Science,* Harcourt, Brace & World, New York, 1961.

Neff, Walter Scott: *Work and Human Behavior,* Atherton Press, New York, 1968.

Nursing Development Conference Group: *Concept Formalization in Nursing: Process and Product,* Little, Brown, Boston, 1973.

Nursing Development Conference Group: *Concept Formalization in Nursing, Process and Product,* 2d ed., edited by Dorothea E. Orem, Little, Brown, Boston, 1979.

Orem, Dorothea E.: *Guides for Developing Curriculum for the Education of Practical Nurses,* U.S. Government Printing Office, Washington, D.C., 1959.

———: "Discussion of Paper, Another View of Nursing Care and Quality," by Lydia E. Hall, in K. M. Straub and Kitty S. Parker (eds.), *Continuity of Patient Care: The Role of Nursing,* Catholic University of America Press, Washington, D.C., 1966, pp. 61–66.

———: "Levels of Nursing Education and Practice," paper presented to the Alumnae Association of the Johns Hopkins Hospital School of Nursing, October 12, 1968, *The Alumnae Magazine,* vol. 68, March 1969, pp. 2–6.

Parsons, Talcott, Robert F. Bales, and Edward A. Shils: *Working Papers in the Theory of Action,* Free Press, Glencoe, Ill., 1953.

Paul, Benjamin David (ed.): *Health, Culture, and Community: Case Studies of Public Reactions to Health Programs,* Russell Sage Foundation, New York, 1955.

Roberts, Mary M.: *American Nursing,* Macmillan, New York, 1954.

Self-Organizing Systems: Proceedings of an Interdisciplinary Conference, May 5 and 6, 1959: edited by Marshall C. Yovits and Scott Cameron, Pergamon Press, New York, 1960.

Selye, Hans: *In Vivo: The Case for Supramolecular Biology*, Liveright Publishing, New York, 1967.

Sigerist, Henry Ernest: *Civilization and Disease*, University of Chicago Press, Chicago, 1962.

Solomon, David N.: "Sociological Perspectives on Occupations," in Howard S. Becker et al. (eds.), *Institutions and the Person*, Aldine, Chicago, 1968.

Somers, Herman Miles, and Anne Ramsay Somers: *Medicare and the Hospitals: Issues and Prospects*, The Brookings Institution, Washington, D.C., 1967.

Sorokin, Pitirim Aleksandorvich: *Social and Cultural Dynamics*, rev. and abr., Extending Horizons Books, Boston, 1957.

Spalding, Eugenia K., and Lucille E. Notter: *Professional Nursing*, J. B. Lippincott, Philadelphia, 1970.

Stewart, David A.: *Preface to Empathy*, Philosophical Library, New York, 1956.

Ullman, Montague: "Health Deviations and Behavior," in Dorothea E. Orem and Kitty S. Parker (eds.), *Nursing Content in Preservice Nursing Curriculums*, Catholic University of America Press, Washington, D.C., 1964, pp. 74–76.

U.S. Surgeon General's Consultant Group on Nursing: *Toward Quality in Nursing: Needs and Goals*, Report, Public Health Service, U.S. Department of Health, Education, and Welfare, Washington, D.C., 1963.

van Kaam, Adrian: *The Art of Existential Counseling*, Dimension Books, Wilkes-Barre, Pa., 1966.

Vernon, M.D.: *The Psychology of Perception*, Penguin Books, Baltimore, Md., 1962.

von Bertalanffy, Ludwig: *Robots, Men and Minds: Psychology in the Modern World*, G. Braziller, New York, 1967.

Whipple, Dorothy V.: *Dynamics of Development: Euthenic Pediatrics*, McGraw-Hill, New York, 1966.

Whitehead, Alfred North: "Part Three, Philosophical," *Adventures of Ideas*, New American Library, New York, 1964.

Wiedenbach, Ernestine: *Clinical Nursing, A Helping Art*, Springer, New York, 1964.

Wiener, Norbert: *Cybernetics*, 2d ed., M.I.T. Press, Cambridge, Mass., 1961.

Willig, Sidney: *Nurse's Guide to the Law*, McGraw-Hill, New York, 1970.

Woolsey, Abby Rowland: *A Century of Nursing, with Hints toward the Organization of a Training School, and Florence Nightingale's Historic Letter to the Bellevue School, September 18, 1872*, Putnam, New York, 1950.

Index

Page numbers that appear in italics refer to tables.